ABOUT THE AUTHOR

Under the stage name Seymour Butts, Adam Glasser has directed and produced more than a hundred adult movies that have sold millions of copies. He was also the reality TV show *Family Business*. A single dad, he lives in Los Angeles, USA.

Adam Glasser, aka

SEYMORE BUTTS

Illustrations by

L. D. Grant · Matthew Shultz

ROCK HER WORLD

THE SEX GUIDE FOR THE MODERN MAN

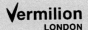
Vermilion
LONDON

1 3 5 7 9 10 8 6 4 2

Published in 2010 by Vermilion, an imprint of Ebury Publishing
First published in the USA by Penguin Group (USA) Inc. in 2009

Ebury Publishing is a Random House Group company

The Random House Group Limited Reg. No. 954009

Addresses for companies within the Random House Group can be found at
www.rbooks.co.uk

A CIP catalogue record for this book is available from the British Library

Penguin Random House is committed to a sustainable future for
our business, our readers and our planet. This book is made from
Forest Stewardship Council® certified paper.

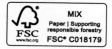

MIX
Paper | Supporting
responsible forestry
FSC® C018179

Printed and bound in Great Britain by Clays Ltd, Elcograf S.p.A.

ISBN 9780091935412

Copies are available at special rates for bulk orders. Contact the sales development
team on 020 7840 8487 for more information.

To buy books by your favourite authors and register for offers, visit.
www.rbooks.co.uk

DISCLAIMER

The stories you are about to read are true. However, some names have been changed to protect the innocent . . . and the not so innocent!

—AG

DEDICATION

This book is dedicated to my family—my mother, **Lila**, my father, **Jerry**, and my sister, **Eve**—for your never-ending, unconditional love and support. To my fiancée, friend, lover, and partner, **Mirna**. To all the fantastic ladies I have had the pleasure of exchanging body fluids with. To all of you who have written the letters and e-mails that inspired me to take on this challenge. And especially to my son, **Brady**, for being the brightest of all lights in my life. Of course, you cannot read this now, but rest assured you will be receiving a copy on your eighteenth birthday.

CONTENTS

BOOK III ABOUT SEX

ACKNOWLEDGMENTS

This book would not have been possible without the contributions of the following people:

Star Farhad	*Assistant*
Michael Harriot	*Literary Agent*
David Vigliano	*Literary Agent*
Bill Abrams	*Attorney*
Michael Weiss	*Attorney*

All the fantastic ladies who were kind enough to offer their personal sexual experiences, preferences, and perspectives:

Desi Foxx	Alexandra Cage
Michele Whitworth	Feengrkufs
Dana Green	Tiffiny
Smokey Damage	Nikita K
Destiny	Dana
MCB	Serenity
BA	

And these who provided their expertise and suggestions for my female-friendly adult movie list:

Steve Javors	*Xbiz.com*
Christina	*Aipdaily.com*
Chris	*Xcritic.com*
Stephanie	*Adultdvdtalk.com*

SPECIAL MESSAGE FOR NON-READERS, INTERNET ADDICTS, CHRONIC MASTURBATORS, AND COUCH POTATOES

In case you've received this book as a gift and have absolutely no interest in reading it, I would like to suggest some other ways it may be useful to you:

1. You can use it for a paperweight.
2. You can use it as a doorstop.
3. You can use it as a coaster.
4. You can use it to squash spiders and bugs.
5. You can save yourself some money by rewrapping it and giving it away as a gift.
6. You can use it to break glass in case of emergency.
7. You can place it under a candle to catch the dripping wax.
8. If you're handy with an X-acto knife, you can carve out a few chapters and use it as a stash box.
9. You can keep it by the fireplace and use its pages to keep yourself warm at night.
10. Hell, you can always sell it for at least $10 if you forge my signature on the book and auction it off on eBay. Those of you who would rather avoid prison can always auction it off without my autograph, but you shouldn't expect to get more than $8.75 for it.

Needless to say, this isn't your ordinary book. The person who gave it to you obviously put a lot of thought into selecting it especially for you. Even if you're not a reader, this just may be the most useful gift you've ever gotten! Now, thank your lucky stars that you have someone in your life who loves you enough to give you such an extraordinary gift and get back to the more pressing matters you are faced with—like finding hand lotion.

INTRODUCTION

I learned long ago never to assume things or else, as my fourth-grade teacher would constantly tell me, I risked making an "ass" out of "u" and "me." I think it would be naive of me to assume I am so well-known to the mainstream public that anyone picking this book up would automatically be familiar with my name(s)—either one of them. Considering I'm offering advice on the most intimate subjects, I thought it would be appropriate to take a moment to introduce myself and give you a brief history of both Adam and Seymore:

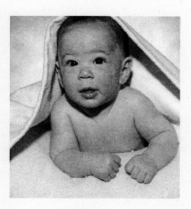

1964-I was born in New York.

1975-Moved to Santa Monica, California.

1978-Lost my virginity to a girl named Jennifer. The entire experience lasted less than two minutes.

1978-The day after losing my virginity, I discovered masturbation.

1980-Got my first job as a "carny" on the Santa Monica Pier.

1980-My first threesome with two girls.

1981-Caught my first STD—venereal warts.

1982-Graduated from Santa Monica High School.

1983-Worked as a shoe salesman.

1985-Graduated personal trainer program at American College of Sports Medicine.

1987-Attended first swing party.

1988-Opened up gym in downtown Los Angeles.

1990-John Stagliano rented out my gym to film a movie called *Where the Girls Sweat.*

1991-I sold my gym and decided to pursue a career in the adult industry.

1991-I shot my first adult movie, called *Street Fantasies,* which featured a girl picking up a homeless guy and fucking him on top of his cardboard box.

1991-I adopted the stage name Seymore Butts.

1992-*The Adventures of Seymore Butts* was released.

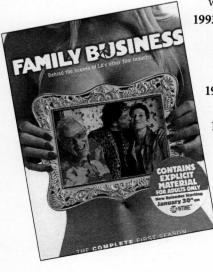

1993-Arrested during adult industry fund-raiser at the Pure Pleasure Bookstore in Las Vegas. No charges were ever filed.

1993-Caught my second STD—herpes.

1994-Misdiagnosis of a skin condition on my penis leaves me with a "spotted dick" (not the kind served in English restaurants!).

1995-Arrested in Florence, Italy, for taking nude pictures of a girl in public. The case is still pending and I'm told I will be arrested if I attempt to enter the country.

1996-My son was born!

1997-My first Web site, seymorebutts .com, was launched.

1998-Won AVN Award for Gonzo Series of the Year.

1999-Won AVN Award for Gonzo Series of the Year.

1999-Arrested in Brussels, Belgium, for taking nude pictures of a girl in public. No charges were filed.

2000-Hired to write sexual advice column for U.K. *Penthouse* magazine.

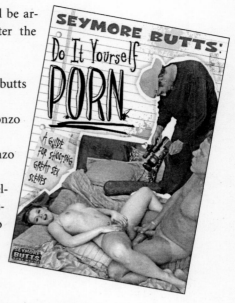

2000-Prosecuted for obscenity by the city of Los Angeles. All obscenity charges were eventually dropped, eighteen months later.

2002-Production of reality TV series *Family Business* for Showtime commenced. The show ran for four seasons in the United States and still plays around the world to this day.

2004-Elected to serve as a member of the board of directors for the Free Speech Coalition.

2005-Inducted into the AVN Hall of Fame.

2006-Inducted into the X-Rated Critics Organization Hall of Fame.

2007-Inducted into the NightMoves Awards Hall of Fame.

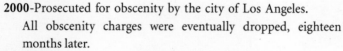

The AVN (ADULT VIDEO NEWS) AWARDS is an annual event that takes place every January in Las Vegas, Nevada. This awards ceremony attracts hundreds of the adult industry's biggest stars and is considered the industry's version of the "Oscars."

2008-Signed publishing deal with Gotham Books to write a sexual advice book specifically for men: *Rock Her World*.

2009-My first site for cell phones was launched, sbutts.mobi.

You should also know that I have had sex with over six hundred women (I stopped counting at age thirty-two) in my lifetime and I would estimate at least 85 percent of those encounters have happened off-camera. I have made over 140 movies during my eighteen-year career in the adult entertainment industry. I am most proud of the instructional movies I have produced, including *Female Ejaculation: A Complete Guide, How to Eat Pussy Like a Champ,* and *Do-It-Yourself Porn.*

After a seven-year custody battle, I was awarded 100 percent physical and legal custody of my son. Currently, we live together along with my fiancée in California. I have been monogamous for the last five years, the longest stretch of one-woman sex I've experienced since I was a teenager! And by the way, I am completely 100 percent satisfied sexually in the relationship I have with Mirna. I believe communication, sacrifice, and mutual respect are the keys to the success of our relationship in the bedroom and beyond its borders. It hasn't always been smooth sailing, but over time we have learned to talk about what we like and need sexually. We have learned that there are times we need to be there sexually for each

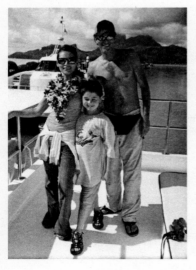

other even if it doesn't "fit into the schedule" or one of us doesn't happen to be "in the mood." Most importantly, we have learned to respect each other's boundaries and not to judge each other for our sexual likes or dislikes, and we both realize our relationship must always travel along a two-lane highway as opposed to a one-way street. In our case, we prefer to call the route the Hershey Highway. Yes, we now share a mutual passion for anal sex, among other things. It wasn't always that way, though. When Mirna and I first began dating, she felt it necessary to tell me that her ass was an exit-only orifice. With patience and a plan, Mirna was soon as enthusiastic about anal sex as I was! You can read more about these techniques in the chapters that follow.

Now I need to backtrack for a moment. I want to discuss that "six hundred" number for a moment. Some of you may read that I have slept with over six hundred women and say to yourselves, "That lucky motherfucker!" I would have agreed with you up until my middle thirties, but now I don't consider the number of sexual encounters I've had to be anything more than an indication of my intimacy issues, and that I'm a great liar! Let's face it, in order to bed over six hundred women you've got to be willing to say or do anything it takes to achieve your goal—whether you really mean it or not. I wasn't able to gain this new perspective until I looked back into my adolescent years to examine the origins of my "physical sexuality." It didn't take me long to realize the root of my intimacy issues—I always seemed to find a physical flaw on a woman that I was always able to use as justification for moving on to the next woman. You see, even though I had intercourse before discovering masturbation, I spent much more time as a teenager having sex with my right hand than with women. At that time, it was Betamax videocassettes and magazines that I masturbated to. When I look back I see how the masturbation patterns of my early years morphed into the relationship patterns of my later years. If I didn't like something about the girl, I turned the page or hit the fast-forward button—just like I did with real women in real life! I have no doubt my experiences meeting these "fantasy girl" types through my career in the adult industry helped me see the light—their shit stinks just like mine and yours. There are no perfect fantasy girls out there waiting for you to ride up on your white horse. This was something I needed to realize before I was able to have a healthy, monogamous relationship with one woman. If I ever find myself reverting to old thought patterns, I remind myself of my sexual roots and then go stand in front of a mirror naked and give thanks for the woman who loves me despite my flat ass and flamingo legs!

Okay, now that you know more about me than my own mother, let me give you an idea of why I decided to write this book and who I wrote it for. I have received tens of thousands of letters and e-mails over the course of my career from both men and women asking for sexual advice. While the men asked many questions about their own performance and how it could be improved to better satisfy their partners, the women were asking me how they could get their men to be better lovers. It didn't take me long to figure out that 2+2=69 and there was a need for a book like this.

Yes, this is a book for men. It's about more than how to be a great lover. My goal is to help today's sexually active men (and those desiring to become more sexually active) not only survive, but thrive in this new millennium filled with hypocrisy and contradiction and bound by a set of ambiguous new rules. Let's face it, gentlemen, the times, they are a-changing! Between the media, women, and the competitive nature of man, there is more pressure placed on men to excel sexually and romantically than ever before. The fact is, male and female sexual behaviors are becoming increasingly similar. Women are much more comfortable today, even encouraged to discuss their sexual conquests, desires, and fantasies, and the sexual prowess of their lovers—with other women and especially in the media.

Women are now becoming empowered through their sexuality and it is up to you as a man to keep yourself in the game. Refining your sexual skills is certainly a step in the right direction, and I will go into great depth to help you achieve this. However, to me, the quickest way to become a legitimate "player" whom women are drawn to, whom women can give their respect and admiration to—something they naturally crave giving their man—is through the acquisition of knowledge. In my opinion, this is the only way for men to combat this change in sexual behavioral patterns (which is most certainly a psychological reaction by women to centuries of male dominance in and outside the bedroom, combined with the rise of the gay community and the recent emergence of the metrosexual). You really can't blame women for wanting to experience the same feelings of power and pleasure that men have enjoyed forever. You can't blame them for feeling neglected and shortchanged sexually. You can't blame them for getting frustrated because they only have orgasms 29 percent of the times they have sex. You can't blame them for not just wanting any man, but wanting "the man." Modern women might talk of enjoying the challenge of "taming" a man, but they still desire a man to be king of their jungle! Literally, there are many women who will go their entire lives without being fucked properly, and I believe it is our duty as men to try to put an end to this injustice . . . can I get an amen!

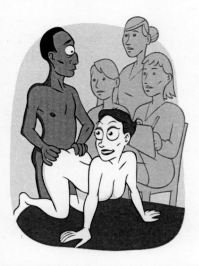

"Oh, don't mind them—those are just my friends,
they're here to judge you."

Instead of laying blame and lamenting societal changes, you need to understand what's happening and educate yourself about women and all things having to do with male/female sexuality. Trying to understand how women think (good luck!) and learning how their bodies work—even more importantly, how your partner thinks and how her body works—is critical. Reading this book is a great start, but you shouldn't consider it an endpoint. Reading "women's magazines" and visiting "women's Web sites," no matter how painful it may sound, is a great way to continue your education and better your understanding. Written by women, specifically for women—can you think of better places to gain insight on women, especially their perspective on men and sexuality?

Your job will be to absorb as much knowledge as possible from this book, as knowledge is the key and common ingredient in the formula for success of the world's most accomplished men, both inside the bedroom and out. The formula is as follows:

Knowledge=power+self-confidence
Power+self-confidence=the ultimate aphrodisiac

Gonzo is a filming style of adult movies that attempts to place the viewer directly into the action. This is accomplished with the extensive use of the POV perspective—the cameraman actually participates in the sex scene while filming or by having the performers communicate directly into the camera to the viewer.

This doesn't just apply to an increase in sexual attention from the opposite sex. When applied to matters of everyday life, it could mean the difference between getting that job you want or not, your ability to close the "big deal" or not, whether or not you get that raise you feel you deserve.

Like I said, this is not just a book about sex, it's about women—listening to what they say and understanding what they want. It's about the human body and how it functions sexually and physiologically. Most importantly, it's about you and how to improve your personal and sexual relationships with women.

I have crammed every bit of pertinent sexual information I have learned over the last thirty years, from the day I lost my virginity, a ninety-second encounter that triggered my voracious sexual appetite and dedicated curiosity, to the day I put the last word to paper in this book. By the time you finish reading that last word, you will be ready to rock any woman's world.

ROCK
HER WORLD

In the beginning, God created Earth and rested.

Then God created man and rested.

Then God created woman. Since then, neither

God nor man has rested.

BOOK I
ABOUT YOU

CHAPTER 1

What's in It for You . . .

'm assuming that's about all the introduction to me any one man could stand, and I'm also assuming some of you might have even speed-read through it, as I realize you may not be used to reading anything without a centerfold and may look at the number of word-filled pages ahead and say to yourself, "Who the fuck has the time to read all that?" I have two things to say to that: One, there are plenty of pictures (I tried to talk the publisher into a centerfold but he didn't bite!), and two, take a look at what you have to gain, in eight short sentences:

1. You will learn how to make yourself more attractive to women.
2. You will learn how to eat pussy like a gourmet.
3. You will learn how to fuck like a rock star.
4. You will learn the secrets of satisfying any woman.
5. You will know what it feels like to be "the man" in a woman's eyes.
6. You will learn how to stoke the fading flames of your relationship into a raging forest fire.
7. You will gain a newfound self-confidence that will benefit you in and beyond the bedroom.
8. You will learn how to navigate through some of life's most difficult and treacherous sexual terrain.

Now, if that doesn't motivate you to lock yourself in a room with this book and not let yourself out until you've finished it, I don't know what will. Wait a second, actually I do have one more idea . . . please flip the page.

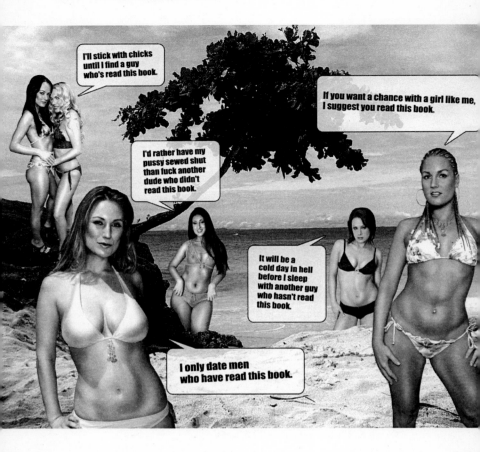

I had a feeling that would do the trick! Now, let's stop wasting time and move on to the important stuff. You will find the following diagrams on the next page: a male sexual anatomy illustration and a female sexual anatomy illustration.

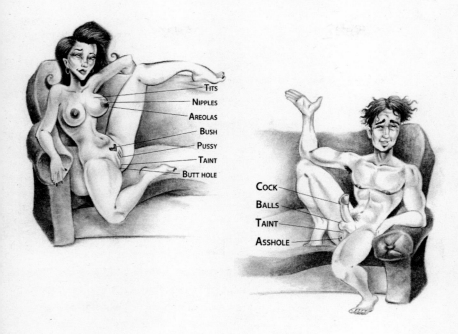

Take a look at the diagrams now, but most importantly, use them to refer to as you continue reading, whenever you feel it necessary.

Obviously, I'm just having some fun! There will be many more detailed diagrams and illustrations for you to refer to when the time is right. Okay, that's really enough of that. Time to get to the serious shit!

CHAPTER 2

Three-Pump Chump

The definition of premature ejaculation is simple: whenever a man reaches orgasm before he wants to. It is estimated that about 40 percent of American men suffer from this problem, but I would be willing to bet that the number is much, much higher in reality. I say that because not only have I witnessed the world's most famous male porn stars struggle with the problem, but I myself have to deal with it from time to time. In most cases, the reason for premature ejaculation is one of two things: overexcitement or anxiety. Personally, overexcitement does me in, as I have occasionally had to really battle against coming quickly when I've gone without sex for four or more days. Some of those battles I've won and some I've lost.

Believe me when I say I know how frustrating and embarrassing being a three-pump chump can be. One of those losing battles that comes to mind immediately occurred during my junior year of high school. I was invited over to a girl named Amy's house to hang out with her and her friend Taren. Amy's mom was at her boyfriend's for the night. Hold on a minute, I think it would help if I give you the backstory of how I met these girls. A few weeks earlier, my friend Tom and I were eating dinner at La Barbera's Pizzeria on Wilshire after working out at the gym. Two hot chicks were already seated and eating when we arrived. Just as Tom and I began to dig into our meals, the girls passed our table on the way to the exit. As they passed Tom blurted out, "Hey, where you two going?" This wasn't unusual for Tom, who wholeheartedly believed in playing the percentages with girls—the more you approach, the more success you are likely to have. I can remember Tom constantly saying, "My grandpa always told me: He who hesitates, masturbates." Anyway, it worked for Tom more often than not, and most importantly, it worked this time! After some small talk, we eventually invited them over to my house because we knew my parents and sister would be asleep by the time we arrived. Thankfully, they were, and we all tiptoed into the guest room to watch TV. Sometime during the next thirty minutes, we paired off—me with Amy and Tom with Taren. Soon after, I asked Amy if she'd like to "see" my bedroom and she nodded with a smile. We closed the guest room door behind us and snuck off to my room. I told her we needed to be quiet because my sister's room was just a wall away. Within seconds, we were dry humping on my bed. After some teenage foreplay, I was on top of Amy, slipping my penis inside of her. She let out a low groan and the rest of the encounter went like this:

Amy: Ooooh . . .
Me: Feels so good . . .
Amy: Ooooooohh . . .
Me: You're so wet . . .
Amy: Oooooooooooooooh! [like a ghost during a haunting and getting loud]
Me: Shhh!
Amy: Ooooooooooooooooooooooh! [louder]
Me: Please, you've got to try to be quiet!
Amy: Oooooooooooooooooooooooooooooooooooooooooooooh! [*too loud!*]
My thirteen-year-old sister (screaming her head off!): Dad, I hear a ghost . . . DAAAAAD!

Let's just say that turned out to be a bad night at the Glasser residence. The next time I talked to Amy, the very friendly ghost, was two weeks later when she called to invite me over to hang out with her and Taren. The moment I walked in the door and saw the girls dressed for a sleepover in sexy little pajama shorts, I knew this was going to be another interesting encounter, especially after I noticed the alcohol on their breath. I declined their offer of a beer but did take a few puffs off the joint they lit up . . . which led to me giving the girls a couple of shotgun hits (inhaling some smoke, pressing your lips against someone else's, and exhaling into their mouth), which led to some kissing, and it was on. I took turns playing tonsil hockey with both Amy and Taren. Soon, all three of us were naked in Amy's mom's bed. They took turns blowing me and I alternated going down on each girl. The girls didn't really interact with each other, but as long as they were both paying attention to me, I was okay with that. Here's the play-by-play of the next few minutes (time references are estimated and for context only):

> 9:30 P.M.-Amy gets on her hands and knees and asks me to fuck her from behind.
>
> 9:30:33 P.M.-I enter Amy from behind and start pumping my cock in and out of her.
>
> 9:31 P.M.-Amy starts moaning like a ghost again.
>
> 9:32 P.M.-Taren tells me, "She likes it when you pull her hair."
>
> 9:33 P.M.-Amy's moans are getting louder and longer.
>
> 9:35 P.M.-Taren, while playing with her own pussy, says, "I love the way she moans like that. It gets me so horny."
>
> 9:36 P.M.-While I'm still fucking Amy from behind, Taren squirms her way underneath Amy, ending up with her mouth directly under my balls.
>
> 9:36:05 P.M.-Taren starts licking my balls.
>
> 9:36:09 P.M.-I come.

I had always fantasized about that particular ball-licking scenario but the reality of it proved to be too much for my nearly seventeen-year-old penis to handle. I was so pissed at myself—and I didn't even get to Taren. I didn't want to admit I came and I made sure to completely internalize my orgasm, so the girls didn't have a clue. Still, I had to think fast. Here's the rest of the call:

> 9:36:15 P.M.-I back away from Amy with a pained expression on my face and my hand on my chest.
>
> 9:36:20 P.M.-Taren, not being able to see my face, says, "Oh goody, my turn."

9:36:22 P.M.-I start acting like I'm having trouble breathing.

9:36:24 P.M.-Amy asks me if I'm okay.

9:36:26 P.M.-I shake my head no and get out the word "asthma" in between gasps for air.

9:37 P.M.-As I struggle to breathe while getting dressed, I tell the girls I'm having a bad asthma attack and need to get home to my inhaler.

9:39 P.M.-I'm driving home cursing myself.

You don't have to be a math whiz to figure out that it took around eight minutes from the time my penis entered Amy to the moment I ran from her house with my tail between my legs. It probably won't be hard for you to believe that was my last encounter with Amy, the very friendly ghost . . . nor did I ever get another shot at Taren. Today, thankfully, I win many more of these battles than I lose because of some techniques I've observed or developed myself over the years. Whether your hair trigger is a result of overexcitement, anxiety, or a bit of both, the aim is always the same—to find a way to control it. Not all of these techniques will work for all of you. However, all you need to do is find *the one* that works best for you.

Masturbation—Or the "spackle before you paint" technique, as my brother likes to call it. Masturbating two to four hours before you anticipate having sex will help some men have a stronger, longer-lasting erection the second go-round.

The Squeeze Technique—When you feel yourself getting close (but not too close!) to orgasm, pull your penis out of her and squeeze it where the head meets the shaft with your thumb and index finger as you very slowly rub the head of your dick over her clitoris. Squeeze for several seconds, until you feel that you've regained control, then continue rubbing her clit for at least twenty seconds before diving back into her pussy.

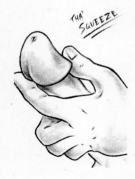

The Stop and Start Method—This is simply a matter of stopping whatever it is you are doing when you feel that orgasm coming on. You can stop and stay inside of her or you can pull out completely. No matter which, you should focus on kissing or eating her pussy at this time. Intimate kissing can be difficult during the throes of passion and this gives you an opportunity to slow things down and concentrate on something else while you regain control. Whether you choose to kiss or eat, she'll be too preoccupied to be thinking about why you stopped. Instead, it will just seem as if it's part of your sexual game plan.

Mind Games—At times, it's just a matter of being able to distract oneself at climatic moments. There are any number of thoughts or techniques a person could use to distract himself. You could set a stroke goal, say fifty or one hundred strokes, and start counting (in your head, of course!) each time your cock moves in and out of her pussy or ass. If you don't feel as if you're in total control by the end of your count, set a new stroke goal and start again. Those of you who are good with numbers might find solving math problems in your head to be extremely helpful. I was once approached by an avid gamer friend seeking advice for the three-pump conundrum and I suggested he try remembering the "cheat codes" to some of his favorite video games when he starts to feel that feeling—he said it worked like a charm! The imagination can also be a powerful tool when it comes to distracting oneself. Try to conjure up images in the mind's eye—images of things that turn you off or disgust you. It could be the image of that asshole of a boss you have or it could be what the asshole of your six-hundred-pound bed-ridden neighbor with the face full of skin tags might look and smell like. Maybe it's the image of a hated ex-girlfriend (as long as she's not naked) or replaying the finale of the "Three girls, two cups, and an electric eel" video you recently watched on the Internet, in your head? Again, it's about finding what works best for distracting yourself, enabling you to regain control before plunging past the point of no return. Hell, I don't care if you to pull out a Rubik's Cube (although she might).

Deep Breathing—Many men have discovered focused, rhythmic deep breathing to be very helpful for maintaining orgasmic control. Not only does it serve as a distraction for the mind, but it also helps to induce a relaxed state. Like the song sings, "Relax, don't do it. When you want to go to it. Relax, don't do it. When you want to come." Obviously, Frankie learned some things in Hollywood because he's absolutely right. Breathe in deeply as you pull out and exhale as you plunge in. Match your breaths to your strokes. Concentrate on feeling your lungs fill up completely and focus on feeling them deflate as you breathe out.

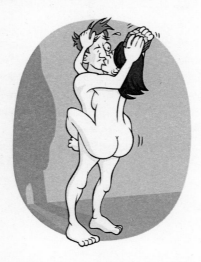

Prostate Exercise—When you feel Old Faithful approaching, stop pumping and do a series of ten repetitions of the prostate exercise called the Piss Off in the section of chapter 4 titled "Sexercise" (page 24). Once you've regained control, start pumping away until you feel that feeling again, then stop and repeat the exercise.

Desensitizing Creams—There are many of these types of products available and they are used successfully by some men. Generally found in cream or spray form, the desensitizing substance is applied to your penis before sex. The substance will have a numbing effect on your cock, causing you to be less sensitive to stimulation and therefore allowing you to last longer. I am not a big fan of these types of products because I feel that sex is all about sensation and I'd rather use other techniques when I'm struggling as opposed to numbing myself completely. The other problem

An average man will ejaculate 7,200 times in his lifetime.

with these products is the risk of numbing your partner's mouth or genitals as the product gets spread around. That's when guys with even the biggest cocks will hear "Are you in yet?"

Dirty Talk—Sometimes all you need is for something to temporarily take your mind off the moment. Talking dirty can do just the trick, especially for men who don't normally do it. Just the process of choosing what words you will say can be enough to distract you sufficiently to regain your control.

Spanking—Again, this is just something else for you to focus on while regaining control. Try concentrating on spanking the fleshiest area of her ass. (More on proper spanking techniques in chapter 23, "Spanking Good Times.")

Increase Frequency—For some men, it's just a matter of getting into a regular, more frequent sexual routine. Making sure you and your partner are having sex at least every forty-eight to seventy-two hours is a good place to start. Of course, I realize this tip is only useful to those with willing partners. Pressuring an unwilling partner into more frequent sex will only lead to other issues. Then again, if you pay attention to what you read in this book, she should be more than willing to have sex with you more often!

Flick and Rip Techniques—First, I'd like to give you a little backstory. As I have mentioned, I have received many letters over the years. One very popular question has always been "How do the male performers in porn last so long when they fuck?" I always answer them with "You can't always believe what you see." The truth is some performers can go forever. They have sex five to ten times per week and have the ability to relax and enjoy themselves. Other performers struggle from the moment their costar puts her hand on their cock. One particular performer I directed on more than one occasion had a very unusual technique for maintaining his control. When he felt himself approaching the point of no return he would either flick his ear or rip the hair off his inner thigh! I have to admit, it was funny as hell to watch. This guy would fold his index finger behind his thumb and literally triple-cock it before unleashing it with furious force against one of his ears. You could hear the snap across the room and my editor would go crazy having to edit the sounds from the audio tracks! When his ears got too sore, he would change things up by placing his hand in position to play with the girl's pussy while he fucked her. Then every so often he would reach for some hairs on his inner thighs, rip them out, quickly toss the hairs aside, and then get his hand back to her pussy. Hence, you have the flick and rip technique!

An average man will ejaculate approximately eighteen quarts of semen, containing over half a trillion sperm, in his life.

Look, premature ejaculation is a very common problem. That being said, you need to remember that it should only be considered a problem if you're not able to last long enough for your partner to get off! Depending on your partner, this could be two minutes or twenty minutes. Keeping that in mind, there is one other way to approach the problem: speeding up your partner's ability to orgasm. That could mean increasing the amount of foreplay or adding a sex toy to the equation. Whichever works best for your partner, it could be a creative and fun solution to your problem.

CHAPTER 3

Mr. Softee

Erectile dysfunction, also known as impotence, is the inability to achieve or maintain an erection sufficient for your or your partner's needs. Although erectile dysfunction happens more frequently in older men, this common problem can occur at any age. Once considered a natural consequence of growing older (decreased testosterone levels) or a psychological issue, impotence is now known to be more often caused by physical problems than by psychological ones. That's why it's not a bad idea to consult a doctor about treatment, because your erectile dysfunction could be caused by a serious underlying medical condition such as heart disease, diabetes, hypertension, or an enlarged prostate. The dysfunction could also be the result of medication you might be taking. These can include antidepressants, antihistamines, antihypertension drugs, diuretics, chemotherapy treatments, Parkinson's disease medications, and hair-growth formulas like Propecia. If the erectile dysfunction is not caused by a physical problem, then the issue lies in your head. These are the most common types of feelings that can lead to a man experiencing erectile dysfunction:

Performance Anxiety—Worrying about whether or not you'll be able to satisfy your partner. This is quite common for men to feel with new lovers.

Physical Anxiety—Concerns about not physically meeting your partner's expectations. Again, this is quite common for men to experience during first encounters.

Stress—When you have so much on your mind that the blood that should be flowing to your penis keeps getting sucked up into your brain.

Depression—You don't need me to tell you what being depressed is like, but I will say that it has the same effect on your erection as stress does.

All right, now that we've talked about the reasons a man may experience erectile dysfunction, it's probably a good time to talk about what he can do about it! There are only a few viable options available, but luckily for modern man, one of them will go down in history as one of the greatest discoveries of the twentieth century: Viagra! Now there are competing drugs available like Levitra and Cialis as well. My answer to any man asking me about treatment for erectile dysfunction is always the same: Go to your doctor and get a prescription for any of the medications I mentioned above. While I have heard that it doesn't work for some men, I have never met any of them personally. I will also let you in on a little secret: At least 90 percent of the men working as performers in adult films use one of those medications every time they perform!

For the men who find those miracle pills don't work for them, there is an even more surefire treatment available, though it does require you to stick a needle in your cock—ouch! It's called Caverject and it is injected into the base of the penis, giving the man an almost instant erection that could last for up to two hours. It's actually been around much longer than Viagra and for a long time was the only option available to X-rated movie studs with limp dicks. After a few months in the business these guys would have cocks that looked like pincushions! Actually, I know some guys who still use it—out of habit, I guess?

"An erection is like the theory of relativity—the more you think about it, the harder it is to get."—Unknown

A man's sex drive is strongest at 8 A.M., but the most popular time for having sex is 10:30 P.M.

Recent studies show that 3 percent of regular male bicycle riders become impotent. This is usually caused by the nose of their bike seat damaging nerves and soft tissue.

Those two treatments are the only ones I can recommend to you based on personal observations or experiences. Although, if the issue is testosterone related, I know great strides are being made with testosterone replacement therapy. There are surgical options available, such as the implantation of vacuum-pump devices, etc., but these should be considered last resorts for a chronic erectile dysfunction problem. I will say that there was a rumor going around the business in the midnineties of a male stud who had one of those vacuum-pump devices installed solely for the purpose of performing in adult movies. It was said that the pump sat in his ball sack and all he had to do to get hard was squeeze his balls a few times. He did work for me on occasion and was an excellent cocksman, so if the rumor was true, the vacuum pumps work well.

Of course, using certain drugs like cocaine, speed, heroin, overconsuming alcohol, or smoking cigarettes could also cause a man to experience difficulties achieving or maintaining an erection. In any of these cases, I highly recommend stopping the consumption of the debilitating substance, as it is likely your sexual performance isn't the only area of your life being affected—if you're doing so much of anything that you can't get hard, it's time to knock it off.

There's one other thing that could be affecting your ability to achieve and maintain erections: excessive masturbation. Let's face it, there are some of you guys out there who are jerkin' their gherkins three times a day or more. That's fine for some of you, but if you're having any kind of erection issues with your partner and are still whacking it multiple

Men who are overweight have twice the chance of being impotent as men of normal weight.

times per day, you can assume you have a compulsion to masturbate and you need to get a grip (no pun intended). Keep yourself busy, try avoiding masturbatory temptation, and save those boners for your partner(s).

The three most common medications linked to erectile dysfunction in males are antidepressants, blood pressure medicines, and sleeping pills.

CHAPTER 4

The P-Spot

The prostate is about the size of a walnut and is located immediately behind the rectal wall approximately one inch inside the anus. Women do not have prostate glands per se, although they do have a G-spot, which is said to be the female equivalent of the prostate. The main job of the prostate gland is to produce semen, the fluid that carries your sperm. The prostate is vital to male sexual function and is considered the man's center of pleasure. It is extremely important for you to be conscious of keeping a healthy prostate, especially as you approach the age of fifty. That's when men, in general, become more susceptible to prostate disease. The three most common forms of prostate disease are noncancerous enlargement, inflammation, and cancer. The scary part of prostate disease is you may or may not have symptoms. That's why it's so important to get your prostate checked by a doctor if you're nearing the midcentury mark. If you did have symptoms of a prostate problem, they could include:

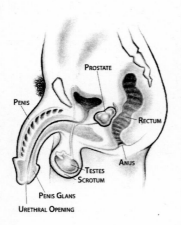

1. Painful urination
2. The urge to urinate often, especially at night
3. Blood in the urine

4. Trouble starting the flow of urine
5. Feeling like your bladder can't fully be emptied

Now, if you're nowhere near the age of fifty and have any of those symptoms, don't freak out, you probably just have gonorrhea! (See chapter 29, "Infection Section," for more info on this.) I am serious, though, when I say every man should get his prostate checked, even you homophobes! Yes, I know I'm suggesting a rectal exam, but I can absolutely guarantee you won't turn into a pickle smoocher. Simply putting a finger up your ass could add years to your life!

Is Assplay Gay?

I am constantly amused by people who believe that a man who is into anal sex with women or having his ass explored by women is somehow secretly gay. Actually, the first experience that I had with this way of thinking wasn't so amusing at the time.

It was June of 1981. I had just barely graduated from eleventh grade and was looking forward to the summer before my senior year. My friends Todd, John, and Lino and I were hanging out in the parking lot of the local twenty-four-hour minimart, as we would usually do before formulating a plan for the rest of the night. It was the place to stop for your liquor, cigarettes, and gum, and it was the perfect place to meet girls and find out about any parties. This was a particularly slow night at the minimart and it also happened to be one of those extremely rare occasions all four of us had some cash to burn in our pockets. After standing around twiddling our dicks for forty-five minutes, the suggestions for the evening's activities began to flow. Bowling, shooting pool, and miniature golf were all met with collective no's. Next, John did something that blew the rest of us away: He came up with a brilliant idea! "What about checking out the new massage parlor over on Wilshire? I heard you can get laid there for thirty bucks!" I don't think I can ever remember all of us piling into the car in such a quick and orderly fashion. No fighting over who sat shotgun; nobody seemed to care all of sudden.

Once we were about halfway to our destination, we all sort of simultaneously realized that none of us had ever been to a massage parlor before. That's when all the speculation began: "Do we pick 'em out of a lineup?"; "Do we pay before or after?"; "Should I tip her?"; "What do I do if her pussy smells?"; etc. By the time we all finished blurting out our questions, John was parallel-parking on Wilshire Boulevard. Lino spoke up: "How fuckin' complicated can it be? We got the money they want and they got the pussy we want. Sounds pretty simple to me!" Lino was a philosopher like that. Then we exited the car and quickly marched single-file through the parlor's front entrance, which was brightly lit by a sign that read #1 ORIENTAL SPA.

We were immediately greeted by a short, middle-aged Asian man who pointed to a sign posted on the wall and explained how things worked. It didn't take us long to realize that John's information was slightly faulty and none of us were getting laid for $30. No, the $30 was the rate to rent your room for a half hour. Once in the room, the girls would explain the massage options and pricing. He did say the massage options ranged in price from $20 to $60. He then led us each to our individual rooms. He ushered me into room number 7 and told me to undress and lay facedown on the massage table. He told me to use the towel to cover my ass and that my girl would be in shortly.

My room was small, probably eight by six, with a massage table, a chair, and a small end table with a lamp on it. The walls were covered with a faux-wood paneling and they were definitely not soundproofed, as I could hear multiple conversations as I lay on the massage table. There was a single oil painting on the wall and the room had a faint yellow glow to it from the dingy shade on the table lamp. It was probably all of four minutes before I heard a dainty knock at the door. It slowly swung open before I could say a word and in walked a pretty enough Asian woman, probably midthirties, wearing a light blue teddy.

"I Jade, what you name?"

"Adam," I said as she moved to the end table, opened the drawer, and pulled out a bottle of lotion. She smiled as she squeezed the lotion into her hands and began to rub them together as she approached me.

"You so handsome!" she said while placing her hands on my upper back. Jade massaged (I didn't realize until later in life that the woman obviously knew nothing about massage) my back for less than ten minutes and then she said, "You go over now."

I had no idea what she meant until she poked me with her finger and motioned for me to roll over. "Now we're getting somewhere!" I thought. She rubbed my chest, stomach, and thighs, casually brushing over my cock as her hands traveled to and fro. The towel that lay over my groin began to look like a tent. Jade quickly noticed she had gained my fully erect attention and smiled slyly again as she asked, "You likey more?"

"More what?" I blurted before realizing what a stupid fucking question that was.

Jade put her finger in her mouth and asked, "You likey?"

"Yes!" I replied.

Jade pointed to her pussy and asked, "You likey?"

"Yes!"

"Forty dolla, one come. Sixty dolla, come two time," she said very matter-of-factly.

You would think I had been given all the information I needed at that point, but no, I had to push it. You see, by that period in my life, I had already started developing my fetish for anal sex. I believe it stemmed from a relationship I had with a heavy-set Greek Orthodox girl whose older sister had convinced her that anal sex didn't count as far as virginity went (I recently met another woman who shares this philosophy, only this one is a porn star who only performs anal scenes for the same reason). Needless to say, my big fat Greek anal sex freak was an exception and not the rule; finding other girls willing to let me drill their derrieres was no easy task for me. Anyway, I figured this was the perfect opportunity to indulge my ever-consuming fetish. So I pointed to Jade's ass and asked, "How muchy?"

She looked at me, puzzled, for a second and asked, "Poo-poo love?"

It took me a moment before I got it. "Yes, poo-poo love!"

Her eyes lit up, unfortunately with fear, not excitement. "Ohhhhhh, you likey poo-poo love, you gay!" She quickly moved away from me and said, "No poo-poo love here," as she flipped a switch on the wall. She then folded her arms and tapped her foot, staring at me as if she were waiting for me to say something.

"Okay, no poo-poo love, no problem! Forget I even asked!"

Jade began to smile again. "You think Jade stupit! You gay, no way! You give Jade AID!"

Now isn't it just my luck to get the Asian hooker who happens to be up on her current events. Earlier in the month, AIDS had been recognized as a serious threat by the world health community. I had no idea what she was talking about at the time, but it was very obviously something she wanted nothing to do with.

Within forty-five seconds of her flipping that switch, the door to the room flew open and a Mount Fuji of a man stood before me. Jade immediately started ranting to him in her native tongue, every once in a while mixing a "poo-poo love" and "he gay" in with the gibberish. He responded to her with one sentence of more gibberish and told me to get dressed. As soon as I had tied my laces, Mount Fuji put a vise lock on my upper arm, escorted me to the front door, and threw me out so forcefully that I stumbled into a parking meter chest-first, which would later result in a bruise that would serve as a reminder of the evening's events for the next two weeks.

I really thought it would only be a matter of seconds before my boys streamed out to lend me a hand, as there was no way they did not hear the commotion through the rice-paper walls! Nope, they were all too busy with fucky/sucky business and at least twenty minutes passed before the last one of my buddies exited, each with a bigger smile than the other. These staggered exits resulted in me having to tell my sad tale three differ-

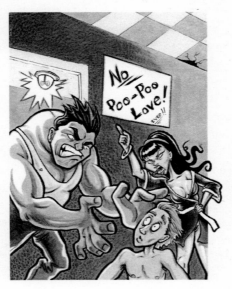

ent times. I could feel the embarrassment factor multiplying exponentially each time I recounted my tragic mistake! That night will be forever remembered, and it is still used to bust my chops to this day. Rarely will my friends and I spend time together when I won't hear one of them whisper in my ear, "You want poo-poo love?"

Now, considering the nature of Jade's profession and the fact that all this happened more than twenty-seven years ago, I can understand her reaction. One would think that with the information available to the public since then, people would have stopped making these types of associations by now. Unfortunately, these perceptions still exist today. That's not to say there aren't many women out there who will not only indulge your anal fetish but find it to be an extreme turn-on! Generally though, even if she finds it to be a turn-on, a woman will wait until you've broached the subject before approaching your nether region or offering up hers. Except for the rarest of situations, you have much more to gain by being honest about your desire for anal sex or prostate pleasure than by staying quiet. Denying or neglecting these desires can lead to pent-up frustrations that can result in impulsive, dangerous behaviors.

Take, for example, the fifty-year-old clergyman from Sheffield, England, who after years of denial became so overwhelmed that he stuck a potato up his ass in an attempt to satisfy his prostate's passion. Unfortunately, he didn't have an exit strategy and quickly realized he would need the help of professionals to extract the spud. He did prove to be a quick thinker, though. To avoid embarrassment, he told the hospital staff it was all just an accident that could have happened to anyone. You see, the clergyman happened to be hanging curtains in the kitchen, naked, when he lost his balance, fell off the stool backward, and landed on the kitchen table—which, of course, had a potato sitting on it. Naturally, the potato became lodged in his anal cavity.

If only we didn't live in a society that was so homophobic! To me, it is a very Neanderthal way of thinking. It's not the sex acts that one enjoys that make one "heterosexual" or "homosexual," it's the gender of the people one desires to engage in these sex acts with that is truly the determining factor. Let's look at it from another perspective. Is it gay for a man with a foot fetish to suck on his ladies' toes? After all, he would be using a similar technique to that of a woman or gay man giving a blow job! Of course it's not gay! The man is sucking on a toe that's connected to a foot, that's connected to a leg, that's connected to a hip, that's connected to a torso with two breasts and a pussy attached to it! If there was a penis attached to that torso it would be a whole other story. It's just that cut-and-dried for me.

Here's one final thing to consider when answering the question at hand: whether assplay is gay. Why was the center of a man's sexual universe buried in his ass if it wasn't meant to be explored? Remember, a healthy prostate is one that is massaged and stimulated regularly. A healthy prostate means firmer, longer-lasting erections and more powerful ejaculations. Prostate stimulation during sexual encounters can lead to super-intense, longer-lasting orgasms. All these fantastic benefits are produced by this walnut-sized gland, and the only way for you or anyone else to reach it is through your ass. It seems very clear to me that anal exploration is part of the divine plan for all males, whether they be heterosexual or homosexual.

Sexercise

Doing exercises that specifically stimulate the prostate will lead to fuller, harder erections and more intense orgasms as well as help keep your prostate healthy while reducing your risk of prostate cancer. Could I possibly make up a better list of reasons? Here are a couple of different exercises and techniques to keep your prostate and your sex life healthy and happy.

The Suck It Up—Stand up and take a few deep breaths. Then exhale until you've expelled all the air out of your lungs. When all the air is out, don't breathe in. Instead, suck your stomach in and up as high as you can into your chest. The "up" part is most important. You can use your hands to help lift in and up. This lifting motion is actually giving the prostate a chance to breathe and stretch out for the moment by removing the weight and pressure of the organs that are piled on top of it, enabling increased blood flow to the area. Now, don't breathe in yet. Pull up some more, as hard as you can. Feel the muscles all the way down to your pubic bone lifting, and while you're at it, give your sides a good squeeze or two as there are many blood vessels located there. It is very important to concentrate on what you are feeling while you are holding your "up and in" position. This process should take ten to fifteen seconds. Then relax, inhale, and rest a minute before repeating the process one more time. This is an exercise that can be done up to three or four times daily and can even be used to combat prostate pain.

Doctors from the Department of Internal Medicine at Bnai Zion Medical Center in Israel have recently declared "rectal massage" as a viable treatment for intractable hiccups.

The Golden Goose—More commonly known as a prostate massage; you can perform this on yourself or take it easy and let your partner do it for you. Fingers, vibrators, and specially designed prostate massaging devices are most commonly used. However, considering the curious nature of humans, I would imagine that just about anything that could possibly fit into an asshole has been experimented with! If you're on your back, the massaging tool should be aimed at an upward angle, and if you're on your hands and knees, a downward angle. Let's imagine you're instructing your partner on how to give you a prostate massage with her fingers, while you're lying on your back and breathing deeply.

First, you instruct her to lubricate her finger and the outside of your asshole with your favorite lubricant.

Then you ask her to place her index or middle finger, palm up, to your asshole and gently insert it until it is all the way in your ass. The depth of the average male prostate varies, but it's usually between two and three inches. It is possible that your partner's fingers may not be able to achieve the depth needed to reach your prostate.

Once her finger is fully inserted, you ask her to apply an upward pressure and start feeling around for a small, walnut-sized protrusion or bump. Tell her to try to aim for the spot where the top of the base of your penis hits your pubic bone.

Once she has located your spot, you ask her to apply a slight pressure to it while sliding her finger back and forth using one-to-one-and-a-half-inch strokes. This stroking action should be repeated five to ten times. After she completes her final finger strokes, you ask her to apply direct pressure to your spot and hold it for a count of ten. You then instruct her to give it a little jiggle before releasing the pressure. Have her relax her finger in your anus for a minute, then ask her to reapply pressure for a final count of ten and one last jiggle. At this point, whether or not you ask her to remove her finger from your ass is completely up to you!

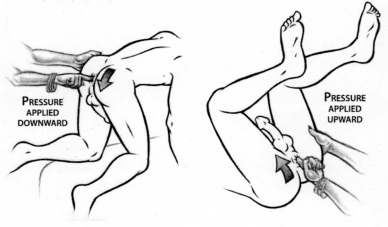

PRESSURE APPLIED DOWNWARD

PRESSURE APPLIED UPWARD

Writing this brings back memories of the first finger in my anus. I was sixteen years old, working a summer job at a shoe store in Westwood, Los Angeles. My manager asked me to drop off a pair of shoes to a lady who lived a few blocks away in a high-rise on Wilshire. Once inside the building, I made my way to the elevators. Five, four, three, two, one—the ding sounded and the elevator doors slid open. An old woman with a walker snailed her way out, followed by a woman with a Chihuahua on a leash. As soon as the Chihuahua laid eyes on me it started yipping. Just as they passed by me, the little turd leaped into the air and latched on to my nut sack. There I was in the lobby of a fancy schmancy building holding a pair of ladies' pumps with a Chihuahua hanging from my crotch, growling at me. First of all it fucking hurt, and second, it was fucking embarrassing. The lady had to hit the dog on the nose a few times before it would let go. "Oh my god, I'm so sorry! I can't believe she did that, it's never happened before. Are you okay?" Before I could really answer, she grabbed me by the arm, led me into the elevator, pushed the up button, and said, "You need to come upstairs with me so I can make sure you're okay. I was studying to be a nurse before I got married." In the elevator, I couldn't help but notice the lady was a fairly attractive brunette—I'd estimate about thirty to thirty-five years old, size 6 to 8, with big breasts. "My name is Diane, by the way," she said as she led me out of the elevator and down the hallway toward her apartment. "I'm Adam," I said, still somewhat stunned by the sack attack. Inside her apartment, she directed me to sit down on the couch, started unbuttoning my pants, and said, "Let's see what we've got here." When my pants and underwear were around my ankles she started examining my twig and berries. There were noticeable bite marks and a slight tear in the skin of my balls. After pointing the marks out to me she said, "I know what you need, I'll be right back," and she disappeared into another room before returning holding a tray with a bowl of soapy water, a washrag, a tube of Neosporin, and a plastic bottle of some sort. Diane then stripped me naked, laid me back, and proceeded to start cleaning my genitals. She was kind enough to throw in a complimentary taint and sphincter wash to boot, and within seconds my injured soldier was standing at full attention. "Don't worry about that," she said. "It's completely normal." I stayed quiet as she started to apply the Neosporin to my wound. When she finished she looked up at me and said, "Okay, now you need to lie back and relax so I can help stimulate the healing process." I realized that plastic bottle contained massage oil as she poured some into her hands. "Just close your eyes and breathe deeply," she said, and I did. I felt her warm, slippery hands take hold of my dick and start slowly rubbing and squeezing it. This certainly wasn't the first hand job I had received, but it was the best. That's what I was thinking to myself until I felt her finger nosing around my asshole. Now, that was a first. I didn't say anything until I felt the pressure from her actually trying to insert that finger. "What are you doing?" "Shhh, just relax and keep breathing deeply. Trust me, this will help you to release your healing powers from within," she replied as she started gripping my cock tighter and stroking it faster—still ever so slowly inching her finger into my virgin ass. It kinda hurt and kinda felt good at the same time. Then she hit a spot with that finger of hers that sent shivers up my spine. She noticed it too, because she said, "There it is," and she continued working both hands like a skilled D.J. Every time I would be on the verge of blowing my load she would stop moving her finger in my ass and squeeze the head of my penis for about ten seconds, only to start stroking and fingering me again. She must have brought me to the edge ten to twelve times, occasionally telling me it was all part of the healing process. Finally, after about thirty minutes she said, "Okay, this time I'm not going to stop. Remember to keep breathing deeply until I'm completely finished." She repositioned herself at my side and she flipped her stroking hand over so her thumb was rubbing the underside of my shaft, concentrating on where the head and shaft meet, while my cock pointed to my chest. The index finger of her other hand continued to poke at my prostate until I was overcome with a rush of pleasure that I can only compare to the feeling of my first-ever orgasm. It was sooooo intense and seemed to last so long, I was shooting come everywhere. Two blasts went flying over my head, the third hit Diane's couch, and the fourth went straight into my eye! I was still coming but I have no idea where the rest of it went, nor could I have cared less as my eyeball was on fire. "Oh, you poor baby!" she said as she led me to the bathroom and told me to wash it out with warm water. Soon the burning stopped but I looked like I had a bad case of pinkeye. After a few final apologies and a kiss on the cheek, I was back in the elevator pushing the lobby button. It wasn't until I started the engine of my car that I realized I had forgotten all about the pumps. Not only had I not delivered them but I left them in Diane's apartment. I just couldn't go back to Diane's and I certainly couldn't go back to work. I pulled over to a pay phone and called my manager, telling her I had been in a car accident on my way to deliver the shoes. I said I would get my car situation straightened out and deliver the shoes on my way to work the next day. Of course, Diane wasn't home when I went to try to pick up the shoes and I'd already bullshitted myself into a corner with my manager, so I decided that my shoe-selling career

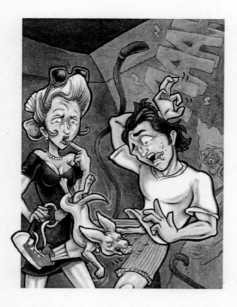

would have to sadly come to an end. I never talked to my manager or walked in the store again. I didn't even collect my last paycheck. Oh, and I never saw Diane again either—but I'll always remember her!

There is another type of exercise that is beneficial to both your health and sexual enjoyment. This one focuses on your urethral sphincter and helps with increased blood flow to your penis and more intense orgasms. This will also help with bladder incontinence problems as well:

The Piss Off—This is about contracting and releasing your urethral sphincter. The first step is to properly identify the muscle group to be exercised. To do this, you'll need to go take a piss. As you begin urinating, try to stop the flow of urine without tensing the muscles of your legs, butt, or abdomen. You should be able to feel the sensation of stopping the stream of urine. Do it a few times. Start pissing (release), stop pissing (contract). Once you've got this down—learned to isolate your urethral sphincter muscle—you are ready to exercise it. I use a combination of three different routines for these purposes. I do mix-and-match sets of rapid-fire sphincter contractions, followed by sets of slow contractions. An example of one of my routines would go like this:

- #1—One set of ten to twenty rapid-fire contractions: Contract and immediately release.
- Rest one minute
- #2—One set of ten to twenty held contractions: Contract and hold for five seconds, then release.
- Rest one minute
- Repeat #1
- Rest one minute
- Repeat #2
- Rest one minute
- Repeat #1
- Rest one minute
- Repeat #2

As with any exercise regimen, you need to continue to add repetitions and increase your contraction hold times gradually each time you do the Piss Off in order to continue to receive the maximum benefits. The great thing about this particular exercise is that it can be done virtually anywhere. You can do it watching TV, talking on the phone, driving in your car, at the office, or even at church. Sometimes while I'm driving and listening to music, I'll try to sync my sphincter up with the beat of a good song. Talk about a workout!

"A sweating ovary or a sick prostate explains most history."
—Martin H. Fischer

Penis Envy

For most men, their issues with the size of their penis are more a matter of perception than reality. Having said that, this is a subject that I will delve into more deeply as you read on. The fact is that whether you really have an abnormally small cock or just think you do, there's really not a damn thing you can do about it. I don't care what those commercials that you see on TV or hear on the radio say. I'm sure most of you are familiar with "Smiling Bob," the guy who sells the pills that are supposed to make your dick bigger. That crooked smile of his isn't due to his cock growing, it's from all the cash he's raking in. That company made millions selling false promises; of course the guy was walking around with a big fuckin' smile! Unfortunately for Smiling Bob and company, their deceptions caught up with them in the form of a federal indictment, resulting in jail time and huge fines. Who's smiling now, Bob? Anyway, the bottom line is there are no pills to take and no amount of pumping or stretching to do that will get you a bigger penis. To be honest, I was starting to think about trying to develop a penis enlargement pill myself, but I decided against it when I realized the financial commitment it would take. Instead, I've decided to wait for someone else to develop the pill and make my millions by opening up rehab centers for men addicted to blowing themselves. In addition to the do-it-yourself enlargement products offered, there are some medical professionals out there claiming to have developed different enlargement techniques, but none of them are endorsed by medical organizations and all have to be considered experimental. I don't know about you, but I don't want anyone experimenting on my schmeckle!

If you're concerned about the size of your cock, you can always learn to more than compensate for it by becoming a master of the oral and digital arts. Learning how to—or refining your ability to—emotionally connect with your partner(s) during your sexual encounters is another way to compensate.

If you won't take my word for it and are still considering a penis enlargement procedure, perhaps you should visit the Russian doctor who is working with special prosthetic penis extension implants like the one he fitted Grigory Toporov with. Unfortunately for Grigory, the extension broke off during a wild sex session with his wife and she has since filed for divorce. Maybe yours won't snap off.

Look, if either you or your partner are absolutely dying to know what it would be like if you had a bigger penis, try a "penis extension" for a bigger-penis experience! You can find a large selection of "penis extensions" at all adult product outlets.

Does Size Matter?

For some reason, the same standard cliché that is applied to houses, cars, boats, and recreational vehicles has found itself being applied to the male penis: "Bigger is better." Unfortunately, over time, the cliché turned to myth and continued to evolve to a point where it is now considered to be fact by many . . . especially those with the big dicks!

Despite popular belief, the truth is, bigger is not necessarily better when it comes to dicks, and, by the way, the same applies for houses, cars, boats, and RVs. I can show you my water, electric, gasoline, gardening, and property tax bills if you don't believe me!

Early man valued penis size as a measure of how deeply he could penetrate his lover, or, simply put, to show how manly he was. Over time, as women became recognized as man's equal and his ability to satisfy her became an issue that was discussed within and outside the relationship, the value placed on penis size became an issue equated with the man's sexual powers. The sexual revolution of the late sixties combined with the continued mainstreaming of adult entertainment from the early seventies to the present day have only helped solidify this "bigger is better" mentality. Yes, there is a small percentage of women—size queens, if you will—who thoroughly enjoy being impaled by a gargantuan penis! It just happens to be a very small number compared to the entire number of females who are sexually active throughout the world.

The average male penis is six inches long and has a circumference of 3½ to 4½ inches. The shortest penis has been measured at 2¼ inches, the longest at a length of 13½ inches, and the thickest at a circumference of 6¼ inches. My penis happens to measure at 6⅞ inches long by 5⅝ inches around. Sorry if that's too much information for you!

There are two ways to measure the length of your penis.

One is done by measuring along the top of the penis, from where the base meets the pubic bone to the tip. The other would be done by measuring along the bottom of the penis, from the tip to where the shaft meets the scrotum. It is widely agreed upon that measuring along the bottom of the penis shaft is not accurate. Today there are products designed specifically to measure the length, circumference, and even volume of a penis. Of course, an old-fashioned tape measure will do the job in a pinch!

No matter how big or small your penis actually is, you need to always remember a few things:

1. The length of the average female's vaginal canal unaroused is three to four inches. When aroused it can lengthen to five inches before penetration. When very aroused the vagina can swell and lengthen to up to eight inches long, but taking a penis this size can stretch it to the point of discomfort for the woman. This is because all women have a cervix (unless it was removed for medical reasons) located at the end of their vaginal canal. The cervix is a delicate organ and most women will tell you it hurts when it's poked by a hard penis!

2. Men and women work differently, especially when it comes to sex and arousal. While men are most tuned in to physical sensation, women are often seeking an emotional connection first and foremost. Since an emotional connection trumps the physical sensation for her, you can see that the size of your penis isn't going to be the thing that determines

whether or not she considers you to be a fantastic lover. No, there are many other factors that shape a woman's opinion of a man's sexual prowess. The difficult part for us men to get is that those factors differ from woman to woman.

3. The G-spot, a key point of stimulation for many women, is located within one to three inches of the vaginal opening. Obviously, it doesn't take lot of length to get to this spot. It's just a matter of knowing where to find it and what to do once you've located it.

4. Don't compare yourself to porn stars! Remember, the guys in porn are in it because of their big dicks and their ability to attain and maintain their erections for long periods of time in the most unusual circumstances . . . not necessarily their sexual prowess. In fact, even the grandiose appearance of the cocks you see in adult movies can be deceiving. Ever heard of the old adage "The camera adds ten pounds"? The fact that you're seeing these dicks on a TV screen makes them appear big. Now add some low camera angles and a wide-angle lens and they look even bigger. Combine all that with the fact that most porn studs shave all or most of their pubic hair in order to make their cocks appear larger and you'll see that you are making unfair comparisons!

5. Looking at your penis from above provides the worst possible view from a size perspective. It's much more impressive to look at a side view in the mirror, or, if you're feeling brave, take a look at the reflection of your erect cock while standing directly over a mirror. That ought to impress you!

6. Sure, having a big cock does have some advantages. You probably love strutting around the locker room naked and you're always the first to suggest some skinny dipping. You're one of the few who looks good in Speedos and women love the way you fill out your jeans. You can get into some sexual positions the less endowed can't, and of course, the size queens love you . . . one time—that is, unless you know what you're doing. Big-dick skills are different than small-dick skills but are a skill set nonetheless. Having a big dick for all to admire is great, but don't think that's all there is to being a great lover or you will end up spend-

ing all your time admiring how big your dick looks in your own hand! One other thing to consider: Size queens aren't born, they are created! Most, probably, by experienced, patient, and considerate men with big dicks. The bottom line is pleasing a woman has very little to do with the size of your penis but everything to do with how well you know your partner, your desire to please, and your technique.

Tipped Off

It is estimated that 40 percent of men worldwide are uncircumcised. If you happen to fall into this category, it is very likely that you have considered circumcision as an adult or at the least wished at one time or another that you were circumcised. This is quite common because of the stigmas that are associated with uncut dicks. First and foremost is the perception of being unclean or dirty. Second, it would seem that women appreciate the way a circumcised penis looks compared to an uncut penis. This is evidenced by two recent surveys:

According to *Psychology Today* magazine, 42 percent of women reported a strong preference for circumcised men, while only 7 percent preferred uncircumcised.

According to *The New York Times*, 81 percent of circumcised men said they had received heterosexual oral sex at some point in their lives, compared with just 61 percent of uncircumcised men.

And now, to top it all off, a recent medical study reports that uncircumcised men are two and a half times more likely to contract HIV from an infected female than circumcised men.

Those broad brushstrokes seem to paint a pretty bleak picture for the uncircumcised. The truth is, if you're conscious of hygiene and safety—as real men are—you shouldn't worry. Just make sure you always keep the following in the back of your mind:

Cosmetic Issues—Uncut men have to take extra care to make sure they keep the foreskin and surrounding areas clean and always conduct a last-minute foreskin inspection before having sex! Regarding the way it looks, trust me when I tell you that if you touch her how she wants to be touched, kiss her how she wants to be kissed, and fuck her the way she wants to be fucked, she won't give a damn what your cock looks like. Besides, you could hit the lottery and hook up with one of those 7 percenters that prefer an uncut cock.

Health Issues—If you are uncircumcised and have a fetish for unprotected sex with strangers or women you hardly know, or men for that matter, then yes—you should probably strongly consider getting that foreskin of yours hacked off! However, if you are a self-respecting man who practices safe sex or is in a monogamous long-term relationship, there is no way I could recommend having the procedure performed, as the potential benefits just don't outweigh the potential for disaster. Now, there are some medical conditions that are best treated with circumcision, in which case, there is no other decision than to do it!

My focus while researching this subject was to find out how men who actually had a choice about being circumcised felt about that choice after the procedure was performed. For me, the guys who did it purely for cosmetic reasons were my target, and here's what I found . . .

I found it's very difficult to find studies on men who elected to have it done for cosmetic purposes as opposed to men who had it done for medical reasons. I did find one study published by *The Journal of Urology*. It included 123 men, 7 percent of whom had the surgery on an elective basis. Of those 123 men, 38 percent felt the procedure caused them more harm than good. That "harm" included erectile dysfunction and/or loss of sensation and sensitivity. That 38 percent seems like a fairly high number to me; however, if that's not enough of a red flag for you, check out some of these quotes I found at Circumcision.org from men who had the procedure as adults:

"I play guitar and my fingers get callused from playing, which is similar to what happened to my penis after circumcision."

"After the circumcision there was a major change. It was like night and day. I lost most sensation. I would give anything to get the feeling back. I would give my house."

"Slowly the area lost its sensitivity, and as it did, I realized I had lost something rather vital. Stimuli that previously aroused ecstasy had relatively little effect."

"After 30 years in the natural state, I allowed myself to be persuaded by a doctor to have the foreskin removed—not because of any problems at the time, but because, in the doctor's view, there might be problems in the future. That was five years ago and I'm sorry I had it done . . . the sensitivity in the glans (penis) has been reduced by at least 50 percent."

As I mentioned, I did find accounts from men who considered their circumcision a success and highly recommended it, but they were too few and far between for me to be able to recommend it. My tip to you is to keep your tip and find yourself a woman who appreciates everything about you, including your uncircumcised penis! Remember, after you're done with this book, you'll have a whole new bag of tricks that are sure to garner you a whole new level of appreciation from the opposite sex.

LATE-BREAKING NEWS ALERT

A man from Louisville, Kentucky, says two doctors amputated his penis without his consent. According to a lawsuit filed in September

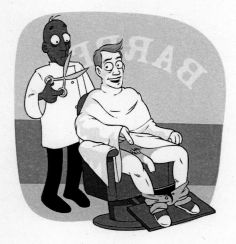

"Just a little off the top."

of 2008, Phillip Seaton went to have a circumcision performed as part of a treatment for a medical condition. Seaton realized his penis had been amputated when he woke up from the procedure. I don't know about you, but I'm more convinced than ever that I should try to avoid letting anyone bring a scalpel within ten feet of my manhood!

There Was a Crooked Man

There are of course no actual bones in your boner. Despite this, it is still possible for you to break your cock. Actually, it's a fairly common occurrence that usually happens when a man is overenthusiastically pumping

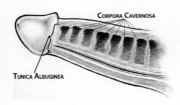

his penis in and out of his partner's pussy and his cock slips out on the out-stroke and smashes against his partner's pubic bone on the in-stroke, causing an audible cracking sound followed by excruciating pain, abrupt loss of erection, and potentially a bent-up dick if not treated by a medical professional. The cracking sound is the tearing of the tunica albuginea, a thick membrane that surrounds the two chambers of spongy tissue that run along the inside length of the penis, called the corpora cavernosa.

Breaking your cock is a medical emergency and must be evaluated and treated immediately. In the most severe cases, it is possible to damage the urethra, interfering with urination. Most often the treatment for a broken penis consists of surgical intervention to repair the tunica albuginea and preserve or restore erectile function and the ability to urinate. Similar to other types of breaks or fractures, the sooner the "broken" part is set, the less likely it is that there will be permanent damage. Left untreated, a broken penis can heal in odd and misshapen ways and result in serious medical problems. In addition, narrowing or shortening of the penis can occur. This condition is called Peyronie's disease. The disease only affects men (of course), is not contagious in any way, and is treatable. It is recommended that you seek treatment from a urologist who specializes in Peyronie's, as the disease and its current treatments are not well understood by some general-practice urologists. Don't let any potential embarrassment keep you from getting treated or you could end up like a porn star I know named Steven, who started performing in my movies in the mid- to late nineties. He was one of the more popular, hardworking studs of the time. All the girls loved working with him—he was young, good-looking, and had a "good dick," as they would say. I'd estimate it was close to eight inches long with above-average thickness and straight as a flagpole. He never had problems with his erection and could basically come on cue—all attributes that made my job as a director and his co-stars' jobs easier. I was disappointed a few years later when I heard Steven had retired to pursue a mainstream acting career. Now fast-forward two years after Steven's retirement. I heard through the grapevine that Steven was back in the biz. I happened to be in the pre-production stage of a movie called *International Tushy,* so I asked my production manager to try to schedule Steven for a scene. Steven arrived on set looking as good as ever. He said he was in the best shape of his life and I believed him. We caught up a bit on old times while we waited for his two female costars, Allura and Mari, to get finished in makeup. After I finished giving the performers and crew their pre-scene pep talk, we began to roll tape. All three nailed their dialogue and transitioned smoothly into the sex. Steven started out by taking turns munching on each girl while occasionally taking a sip from a water bottle and forcefully spitting it at their pussies. It wasn't until the girls started blowing Steven that I noticed something was very different about him. His cock had a dramatic upward curve. When I say dramatic, I mean near-ninety-degree-angle dramatic. And it seemed shorter—at least one and a half to two inches shorter! Despite my desire to yell "cut" and ask him what the fuck happened to his cock, I held my tongue. I didn't want to risk deflating his ego or his cock before we finished shooting the scene, and I knew the girls weren't going to say anything because neither of them had ever worked with Steven before. Thankfully, the scene went off without a hitch and we wrapped after both girls lovingly snowballed Steven's nut butter. Of course, I waited until he was showered up and ready to leave before pulling him aside and asking, "What the fuck happened to your cock?" He explained that he broke it, although he didn't know it when it happened and let it heal on its own. I joked that he should consider getting a tattoo above his pubes that read

"Caution: Dangerous Curve Ahead" but I don't think he appreciated my humor. After he left, both girls made similar comments about the curvature in Steven's cock and the way it felt when he fucked them. Mari actually dubbed his dick "the Spine Scratcher" for the way it felt when she was on her hands and knees while he fucked her in the ass from behind.

Of course, every man with a curved penis didn't necessarily break it and develop Peyronie's disease. There are two other reasons a man might have a curved penis:

Born with It—A moderate degree of curvature of the penis is considered normal, as many men are born with a condition commonly referred to as congenital curvature. This causes the penis to point in a direction (up, down, left, or right) other than straight forward, while still having a relatively straight shaft.

Chordee—A condition considered a birth malformation in which the head of the penis distinctly curves downward or upward. It is best to treat

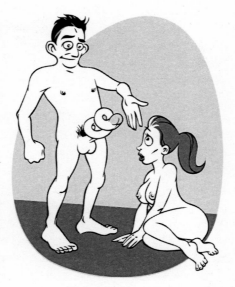

"So that's why they call you
'the sommelier.'"

this condition with surgery during infancy, sometime after the child is six months old and before the child reaches the age of two.

If you think you may have broken your cock or have symptoms of Peyronie's disease, you should consult a doctor immediately. Otherwise, there's not a lot you can do about a curvature in your penis, except make the best of it, of course. While a straight penis has always been seen as the "norm," the fact is, having a slight curve can be an advantage for a man who knows what he's doing and understands female anatomy, as a curved penis could touch spots inside of a woman that a straight one can't. There's much more on this throughout the book, so keep on reading!

What to Do If Your Penis Is Cut Off

Since the day I heard about Lorena Bobbitt taking a pair of scissors to her husband John's penis, I have had a semiregularly recurring nightmare where I suffer the same fate. I always wake up in a cold sweat with my hands on my cock. Maybe I was a little closer to the situation than most— not only did I end up meeting John, but I actually visited the spot where Lorena dumped his dick! Despite the fact that my impression of John was less than positive—he's a total fucking moron—I still can't say I feel he deserved to have his schlong cut off. Lorena did cut it off, however, and that's all that matters for John at this point. Since her snip at fame, other

Three out of every one thousand men are well-endowed enough to fellate themselves to orgasm.

According to condom manufacturers, only 6 percent of men use extra-large condoms.

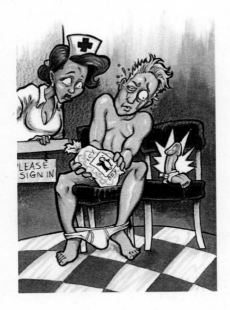

women have followed Lorena's lead. I'm not saying we're in the midst of a cock-clipping, penis-snipping epidemic, but it does happen and you should know what to do—just in case:

Step 1—Scream your fucking head off!

Step 2—Use a towel or something similar to apply pressure to the wound.

Step 3—Call an ambulance and tell them to hurry the fuck up!

Step 4—If you have any semblance of a shaft remaining use a shoestring or something similar as a tourniquet and wrap it around the base of what remains of your dick. Keep applying pressure to the wound.

Step 5—Look around for the rest of your penis. You may be luckier than John and your attacker might have left it instead of taking it for a ride. If you do find it, pack it in ice and put it in a plastic bag.

Step 6—Grab a box of tissues, pray that your insurance is paid up,

In 1609, a doctor named Wecker came across a corpse with two penises. Since then, there have been 80 documented cases of men similarly endowed.

and wait for help to arrive. While you're at it, you might want to cancel her credit card if you can. Studies show that 47 percent of women who have cut off a man's penis go shopping immediately after the incident.

The Family Jewels

There's a reason why your balls are often referred to as the "family jewels": because they're extremely valuable to you and you better protect them like an all-pro offensive line protects their star quarterback. As a young man in my early twenties, I can remember cursing the failure of evolution to provide better protection for my jewels while I lay on the ground writhing in pain after getting hit in the nuts with a nine-iron. Since then I have learned why it is so important that our balls are placed in such a precarious and vulnerable position. Our testicles, the oval masses that sit within a sack called the scrotum, actually produce our sperm. In order for the testicles to do this, they must maintain a temperature 2°F lower than the rest of the body. That is why they must be situated externally and that is why men are told not to wear tight underwear around the times they are trying impregnate their partners . . .

Tight=Friction=Heat.

Cracked Nuts

Now let's go over some of the more common problems a man can have with his testicles.

Testicular Cancer—This will produce a painless swelling of one testicle. It is the most common cancer in young men between the ages of fifteen and thirty-five. The only good news here is that doctors have now achieved a 96 percent cure rate against this form of cancer. Of course, the earlier it is detected, the better the chances of successful treatment. It is recommended every man eighteen and over be checked for testicular cancer once per year.

Infection—The testicles are susceptible to bacterial infection. This is most commonly caused by microorganisms descending into them from the urinary system. When your testicles are infected they will become swollen, tender, and hot to the touch. Infections are generally easily treated with antibiotics, although if left untreated they can lead to infertility.

Testicular Torsion—For stability, the testicles are attached to the scrotum by tether-like arteries that carry blood to them. Testicular torsion occurs when the tethers get twisted to the point of cutting off the blood supply to one of the testicles from above. This will cause serious pain and swelling. Unfortunately, that's not the worst part. If the condition doesn't correct itself or isn't corrected by a doctor within six hours, gangrene will set in and the affected testicle will have to be removed. The only silver lining to that dark cloud is that a man can perform sexually and even father children as long as he has one working testicle.

Kicked in the Balls—Unless you're one of those "bubble boys," you've probably experienced this. Usually, being kicked or hit in the nuts won't cause permanent damage. In these cases, painkillers and a warm bath along with wearing supportive underwear should provide the bruised bollocks with some welcome relief. It is possible that a severe blow could cause testicular rupture. This occurs when blood flows into the scrotum, causing acute pain, extreme swelling, and discoloration. In these cases, it is advisable to get to a doctor as soon as possible.

Most men have one testicle that hangs lower than the other just as most women have one breast that is larger than the other.

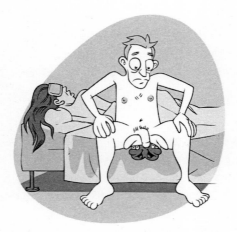

"Oh, please. 'Blue Balls' is a myth."

Blue Balls—Some feminists will tell you that blue balls are simply a ploy devised by men to guilt or pressure women into having sex or getting them off. I certainly won't dispute the fact that many men have used the ruse of blue balls for that very purpose, but that doesn't mean that blue balls isn't a genuine condition experienced by many men. "Blue balls" is actually a slang term referring to testicular pain. When a man becomes sexually excited the arteries carrying blood to the genital area swell, while the veins carrying blood from the genital area become more constricted. This unbalanced blood flow causes an increase in the volume of blood and causes the penis to become erect and the testicles to become engorged with blood. The longer you stay aroused, the longer the blood stays there. Newer blood is red, but older blood is a dark red/purple because it contains less oxygen. As the older, darker blood settles in the testicles over time, it tends to make the skin of the scrotum appear to have a bluish tinge. When the man achieves orgasm and ejaculates, the veins and arteries return to their normal size, the amount of blood in the genital area is reduced, and the penis and testicles return to their usual dimensions rather abruptly. If ejaculation does not occur, causing the blood to remain in the genitals for an extended period of time, there may be a lingering heaviness, aching, or even pain in the testicles. While it may be uncomfortable, blue balls is a temporary condition that will dissipate with the passage of time. Masturbation is also a viable solution that tends to speed the recovery process. If you're one of those guys I spoke of who have used a condition like blue balls to pressure a woman to proceed with sex, whether you had it or not, make sure it's the last time you do it! Besides, once you're finished reading this book, you won't need to use excuses or ploys to pressure women into sex anymore—though you might need to come up with some in order to *not* have sex when she can't get enough of you and your cock feels like it's gonna fall off if you don't get some rest!

CHAPTER 7

Flavor of Love

Women will tell you that all men taste different—their semen, that is. Actually, many women will tell you that, like ice cream, semen comes in many flavors. Ranging from yummy to yucky, the various flavors of semen have become a point of interest and discussion among today's women, especially those who enjoy performing oral sex. If you think about it, how you taste should be something you consider. After all, common sense dictates that if you taste good, your partner will want to eat you more often. So, what can you do to make yourself taste better? Well, first you have to understand that the flavor of your semen will be dictated by what you consume. Yes, it's true: You are what you eat.

Now, let's take a look at a few of the things you might be eating or drinking and how they might be affecting your own "flavor of love" . . .

BAD CHOICES

- Meats and fish—These alkaline-based foods can produce a foul buttery/fishy taste.
- Dairy products—These contain a high bacterial level and can produce a flavor that's been likened to sour milk mixed with old tuna fish.
- Chemically processed liquors—These might make you feel good but they will make your semen taste like rancid lemon juice.
- Asparagus—For some reason, there is nothing, I repeat nothing, that can make your sperm taste worse than a side order of

asparagus. Broccoli and cauliflower can also cause some offensive-tasting semen. You vegetarians should be paying special attention to this. Now you know why you never get a second blow job!

- Curry, garlic, and onions—These should also be consumed in moderation. Eating too much of any of them will not only make your sweet cream bitter but could cause it to have an odor similar to what you might find in the bathroom of a cheap all-you-can-eat Indian restaurant.
- Junk food—Foods loaded with artificial flavorings, colorings, and preservatives will have your man milk tasting like moldy gouda cheese.

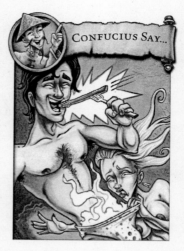

Man who eat asparagus
have bad taste in
underwear

GOOD CHOICES

- Cinnamon
- Cardamom
- Peppermint
- Lemon
- Parsley
- Wheatgrass
- Celery
- Acidic fruits and juices
- Naturally fermented alcohol
- Zinc/selenium supplements

All of the above can give your semen a pleasant sugary flavor. Drinking plenty of water will also help rid the body of toxins, which will lead to fresher-tasting sperm. My personal semen sweetener of choice is pineapple juice. I've been told I taste sweet and fruity after drinking a couple of glasses each day.

"If God was a woman she would have made sperm taste like chocolate."—Carrie P. Snow

CHAPTER 8

Typecasting

A man's sexual attitudes and behaviors offer great insight into the man as a whole. Men have traditionally fallen into one of the following groups: heterosexual, homosexual, and asexual. During the sixties and seventies a new group gained mainstream acceptance in the fertile valley existing between heterosexuals and homosexuals: bisexuals. Through the nineties and now at the turn of another century, men are being offered even more micro-niched terms to define themselves by. Men who previously defined themselves as "normal" heterosexuals have now been divided into two subgenres—metrosexuals and retrosexuals. A metrosexual is defined as a male with a heterosexual orientation who rejects many macho attributes often linked to masculinity. He has a strong aesthetic sense and spends a substantial amount of time and money on his appearance and lifestyle. A retrosexual is defined as a male who spends as little time and money as possible on his appearance and believes in traditional roles for men and women. Personally, I don't see myself fitting in either category, and you might be having the same problem. In an effort to provide like-minded guys with a term to identify with—a group to belong to—I have coined the term "dynosexual." Dynosexuals are defined by me as males with a variety of interests and skills, sharing the single common-

"In the animal kingdom, the rule is, eat or be eaten;
In the human kingdom, define or be defined."—Thomas Szasz

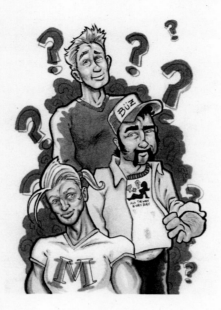

ality of extensive sexual knowledge and abilities, along with the desire and willingness to explore all paths that may lead to total sexual fulfillment for both their partners and themselves. Considering we are just getting started on this journey together, it's a good time for you to start thinking about these kinds of things.

"Pathetic attitudes are not in keeping with greatness."
—Friedrich Nietzsche

	METROSEXUAL	RETROSEXUAL	DYNOSEXUAL
Sports Interests	Loves to golf because of the great outfits he gets to wear. Watches soccer to see how Beckham is styling his hair.	He's into the four major sports, roller derby, and wrestling. Thinks soccer is boring and golf and tennis are for pussies.	Appreciates all sports for the skill they require, just as he appreciates all women for their individuality.
Buying Feminine Hygiene Products	He has no problem going because he needs to pick up some hand cream.	Will go to buy under protest if he thinks he won't get laid for the next two weeks if he doesn't.	Has no problem with it and doesn't mind fucking his partner when she's on her period either, as long as she's into it.
His Drink	Lychee martini.	Beer and a shot of whiskey.	Absinthe.
Buying Drinks	He'll buy if he has to but would prefer to go dutch.	He'll keep buying as long as she keeps drinking. He sees alcohol as a tool to take advantage of women sexually.	He has no problem buying and doesn't expect anything in return. If he sees the woman might be drinking too much he'll politely say something to her.
Cunnilingus (Eating Pussy)	He might or might not, depending on his mood. If he's having a bad hair day, forget about it!	Feels it's a man's way of having to make up for a small penis.	Will do it any time because he knows his partner loves it.
Getting Kinky	As long as the girl is gentle and doesn't leave marks.	As long as it doesn't include his ass or anything that might make him look like a turd burglar.	Gets kinky with the best of them. Has the knowledge and skills to adapt to a variety of sexual environments and activities.
Finding the G-Spot	He can find it but doesn't want to worry about having his new Egyptian cotton sheets ruined.	He works hard enough all day; he doesn't have the energy or the inclination to start looking for anything during sex. Besides, what does he get out of it?	He knows exactly where to find it and exactly what to do with it to rock her world!

	METROSEXUAL	RETROSEXUAL	DYNOSEXUAL
Getting Manicures and Pedicures	Gets them because he thinks they make his hands and feet look nice.	Men have lived for thousands of years without washing their hands every fifteen minutes. Why start now? Manicures are for knob gobblers anyway.	Gets them because he doesn't want to hurt his partner while he's fingering her to orgasm.
Physical Abuse	Not likely; he'd be worried about getting an ugly bruise if things got physical.	Only when she deserves it.	Absolutely never.
Things You'll Find in His Refrigerator	Depends on what diet he's on that week.	Beer, leftovers, TV dinners (Hungry Man).	Wine, strawberries, whipped cream, pineapple juice, and some cucumbers and zucchinis just in case his date has a veggie fetish.
Things You'll Find in His Nightstand	Eye mask Picture of himself Hairnet Condoms	Jar of Vaseline Loaded gun No condoms, because birth control is the chick's problem	Lubricant Incense New vibrator Extra batteries Condoms
Things You'll Find in His Closet	Custom dress shoes with built-in lifts Linen pants Sandals Bow tie	Army boots Full camouflage gear Tie with mud-flap girl print	Tux Alligator shoes Flip-flops
Underwear	Thongs or briefs with padded butts.	Boxers with mud-flap girl print.	Boxer briefs.

CHAPTER 9

Lust vs. Love

Love is such a crazy thing, yet it is only just a word. Being in love can mean many things to many different people, which makes the whole concept of being in love a confusing one, at the least, for many of us. More often than not, we confuse infatuation or lust with love. There are some of us men who think we've found the "one" because we didn't want to leave her the second we finished ejaculating, but what we fail to realize is it's just a case of being sexually compatible, as opposed to falling in love. Being sexually compatible is not a true indication of being in love. There are many couples in this world who actually hate each other outside of the bedroom but are still able to make the magic happen for each other inside it. Some think their desire to bring a girl home to meet the parents is an indication of having "special feelings" for her, and yes, while that could be true, it could also just simply be a way for a man to show off or get approval from his parents (especially his father) in a "look at the piece of ass your son's banging now" kinda way. Some guys will convince themselves they're in love with the first girl who spreads her legs for them, while others will let themselves be convinced of it due to pressure placed by overbearing partners. For those of you who find it difficult to determine the difference between being in love and being in lust, I have put together a list of true-love indicators that will hopefully help clear things up for you now or in the future:

"Sex without love is merely healthy exercise."—Robert Heinlein

"Love is the self-delusion we manufacture to justify the trouble we take to have sex."—Dan Greenburg

TRUE-LOVE INDICATORS

1. When you look at her, do you get more than just the "I wanna fuck that" feeling? Do you find yourself genuinely caring about her happiness, well-being, and success?
2. Do you feel truly happy and satisfied when you wake up next to her in the morning? I can hear some of you now: "Sure, when she wakes me up with a blow job!" By now you should know that's not what I'm talking about! I'm talking about an over-whelming "it's good to be alive" kinda feeling.
3. It is natural for thoughts of cheating to creep into every man's mind at one time or another, but there are those of us who know deep down that we could never do it because of the pain and damage that it could potentially bring to our partner and relationship. Do you feel this way?

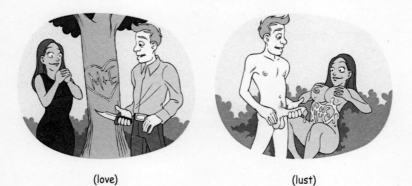

(love) (lust)

4. Do you feel like you can tell her anything—even your deepest, darkest secrets?

5. Whether or not you are the type of man who has the ability to compartmentalize his feelings and emotions, do you find yourself thinking about her at unexpected times? Do you imagine what it would be like to grow old together?

6. Are you really interested in hearing her speak about her dreams and ambitions? About the time she threw up at band camp or that she wanted to be an astronaut when she grew up? Some of us will pretend to enjoy this banter because we think it's the path of least resistance to getting laid.

7. Whether you're making plans for the short-term or long-term future, do you find yourself considering the effects these plans may have on her and your relationship first and foremost?

8. Do you have a desire to learn about or experience things that she enjoys?

If you answered no to any of the questions above, I have no doubt you're in something—but it's probably not love. However, if you answered a resounding yes to all—consider yourself a lucky man, because you probably have found the one! Let's just hope she feels the same way about you!

Studies show that events that occur in the brain when you're in love are very similar to those that are found in people who suffer from obsessive-compulsive disorder.

"Love is a condition in which the happiness of another person is essential to your own."—Robert Heinlein

CHAPTER 10

Cheaters Never Prosper

I have to be honest and admit I have cheated quite a few times in my relationships of the past, starting my indiscretions at the tender age of seventeen. Proudly, that type of behavior is behind me. The last time I was unfaithful was the last time for a reason—I almost got killed! I had been dating Misty, a statuesque brunette personal trainer with Maria Sharapova legs and a world-class ass, for about two and a half years, since I was twenty-six. Being a personal trainer myself, I decided it would be a good idea to open up a "boutique" gym in downtown Los Angeles. Equipping the gym was crucial and had me dealing with vendors and sales reps all across the United States. There was one particular sales rep who eventually came to stand out above all the rest—the woman selling me a spring-loaded aerobics floor. Her name was Holly and the first thing that I noticed was her voice. She spoke softly, with a slight rasp, but it was more the tone and the way she spoke—I can only describe it as eargasmic! It was all very innocent at first. After all, she lived on the other side of the country. I don't know exactly when it happened, but sometime after the first couple of business-only calls, pleasure got mixed into the equation. First, it was double entendres like:

Me: How do you treat the wood?
Holly: I worship it, especially if it's hardwood!

The next thing you know our conversations were more aural sex than floor specs. Again, while I knew these types of conversations wouldn't be appreciated by Misty, I really didn't think anything would ever come of them because of Holly's geographically undesirable location. That is, until quite a few months after the gym's grand opening, when I got a call from Holly telling me she had to come to Los Angeles for business and she would be staying at a hotel less than ten miles away from me. I suggested she visit the gym, she suggested we have dinner—I should have known then that this was leading to trouble. Of course, my curiosity got the better of me—which, as I now look back, can safely be attributed to four main factors:

Factor 1—I was weak.

Factor 2—Her voice.

Factor 3—During one of our phone conversations Holly described herself as a petite (five foot two) natural redhead with a gymnast's body. I always had a thing for Nadia Comaneci and had never been with a natural redhead.

Factor 4—Probably the single biggest factor: One of our conversations had gone something like this . . .

Holly: Can I ask you something?

Me: Sure.

Holly: Promise you won't think I'm weird or a freak?

Me: Promise.

Holly: What do you think about anal sex?

Me: Are you serious?

Holly: I knew it. Forget I asked!

Me: No, I meant that in a good way. I am totally into it!

Holly: Me too! It's my favorite. I just haven't met a lot of guys that are really into it.

Can you really blame me? Don't answer that—of course you can blame me; I blame myself. What I did wasn't right even if running into a girl like Holly is a dream come true for an anal sex freak like myself. Anyway, here was the plan . . . I would tell Misty I was going to dinner with an equipment sales rep. I would pick Holly up for dinner at seven thirty and then swing her by the gym, which would be closed by then, before dropping her back off at her hotel. We didn't make it to dinner or the gym—we didn't even make it out of her room. She exceeded even my most optimistic expectations. Much cuter than a button; tight, compact body; and the red hair—she described herself perfectly. I have to assume I at least met her expectations, because it wasn't three minutes after her door closed behind me that I was buck naked and literally ripping the button-up blouse off of her. We were two of a kind. We might not have made it to the restaurant but that didn't stop her from ordering up some stuffed sphincter with a side of ass à la mode or either of us from eating plenty of brown-eye pie. For our final course, it was hot loads of sweet cream in Holly's hot buns as she screamed with delight.

I made it home that night by close to one A.M. to find Misty fast asleep. In the morning, everything was business as usual. If only I could have been satisfied with my one night with Holly. I should have just declined when Holly called on Sunday morning asking if I had time to show her the gym that afternoon. Instead I told Misty that a friend called at the last minute with an extra ticket to the Dodgers game. After I picked Holly up, we arrived at the gym around one P.M. As usual, the gym was closed on Sundays because we catered to people who worked downtown—so we had the place to ourselves. I gave her a quick tour of the facility and she took a few pictures of the aerobics area before excusing herself to use the restroom. When she exited five minutes later, she was naked save for ankle socks and tennis shoes, saying, "I want to make sure your floor was installed properly. Can you put on some music for me?" So I hit her with some Neneh Cherry as she pounded on my floor. When the song was over she exclaimed, "It was installed perfectly!" as she made her way over to the stereo and started searching through our cassette tapes. Soon, Enigma was blasting and Holly was approaching me with that "enough of this pussyfooting around, it's time for a cock in my ass" look. Things heated up fast from that point, both physically and literally. It happened to be a blazing hot day in the dead of August, but I didn't even think about turning on the air-conditioning when we arrived. There we were, sweating like heroin addicts in withdrawal while we did the hokey pokey on my perfectly installed aerobics floor. At least thirty minutes later, Holly was on her haunches as she squatted her buns of steel up and down my love muscle. Sweat was pouring off her, while her breathing became fast and heavy.

"I think I need to take a break," she gasped as she disengaged her butthole from my cock and stood up. Still not able to catch her breath, she squealed, "I think I'm hyper . . . ventilating!" I thought some cold water might help but before I took two steps I heard a loud thud and turned to see Holly sprawled out on my perfectly installed aerobics floor—completely unconscious. First I panicked. Then I tried to revive her. Finally, I called an ambulance. By the time the paramedics arrived, Holly had partially regained consciousness. They diagnosed Holly with a grade 2 concussion and recommended a visit to the hospital, but she declined, instead asking me to take her back to her hotel. She left town the next day. Meanwhile, Misty had to be at the gym early Monday morning to work out a client. When I got in, I found Misty in the office crying. When I asked her what was wrong, she called me a "fucking bastard" and lunged at me with a pair of scissors. Luckily, I was able to catch hold of her wrist and wrestle the weapon away. While I ended up with a small nick on my forearm, it was obvious Misty was the injured party. She ran out of the building and drove straight to our place, where she packed up her possessions and left. Over the course of the next couple of days I was able to piece together the fol-

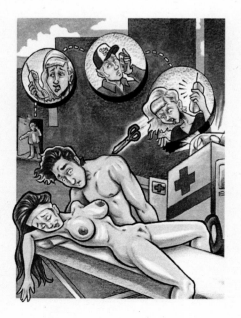

lowing: One of the security guards who worked across from the gym happened to see me talking to the paramedics and mentioned it to Misty. Then she got hold of my friend who I said invited me to the game, and of course he had no idea what she was talking about. The Dodgers weren't even in town! There was absolutely no way I was going to be able to bullshit my way out of this one. Misty had me dead in the water and that's exactly how she left me . . . almost.

I listed the factors that I believe contributed to this particular transgression. It's easy to do in hindsight. I just wish I thought about things then like I do now. If I would have taken some time to think about the reasons I was doing the things I did, I would have saved myself and others from a hell of a lot of stress and heartache. Up until recently, it was believed that, in general, men cheat for sex and women cheat to fill emotional voids. As I have said repeatedly, the times, they are a-changing, and so are the reasons that men and women cheat. The hard facts are, we men are becoming more emotionally driven as a group, or more feminine, if you will, while women are becoming more masculine. The proof is in the pudding. Note the rise of the metrosexual male and the increasing numbers of gay, bisexual, and transgender men and consider that the number of violent crimes committed by women has risen dramatically over the last two decades, that the percentage of women having extramarital affairs has increased exponentially in recent times, and that there continues to be a high amount of discussion and media focus surrounding the sexual satisfaction of females. To me, it seems pretty obvious we are in the midst of a continuous paradigm shift in the traditional male/female roles. Actually, tradition probably left the room in the late sixties and has been on the run ever since. Okay, now that I've beat that bush silly, let me get to

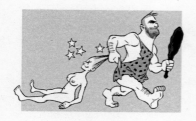 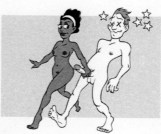

then & now

my point . . . many men think they are cheating for sex or due to a lack thereof, while they are really seeking a type of emotional support or a feeling of appreciation. Whether that means hearing how talented they are at their job, how attractive they are, or what a great lover they are, these kinds of affirmations need to be heard by men. The problem is many women have no clue, mainly because men don't like to admit it and are reluctant to discuss these types of emotional needs for fear of making themselves look "weak" to women, or to other men, for that matter. Hey, it's not like women don't like to talk. Sometimes, it's just a matter of us men clueing them in to the things we'd like to hear. For a woman who loves you and truly values the relationship you have together, this type of request should be readily accepted and complied with. It is not asking a lot! However, if you have repeatedly failed to comply with her similar re-quests in the past, you probably shouldn't expect any request you make to be readily accepted. Women, especially good women, just aren't willing to travel down that one-way relationship street anymore. For the good ones, it's a two-lane highway or nothing . . . preferably the "Hershey Highway," from my perspective! Anyway, as I was saying, many times an issue like this can be solved by initiating a simple discussion like this:

"I need you to do something for me. It would be really nice to hear you say some of those things you used to tell me . . ."

Or:

"You know how you feel when I tell you how sexy you are or what a great job you do taking care of our home? Nothing would make me feel better than hearing those types of things from you . . ."

If you're not comfortable with a conversation, write her a note:

Hey, Baby,

I don't ever want you to forget how much I love you. Of course, I know you love me but I feel like I need to tell you that I would love to hear how you feel about me. I know you think these things aren't important to me, but they are . . . most importantly, the words would be coming from you! Is there anything you need more of from me?

The average man experiences eleven erections every twenty-four hours and has a multitude of sexual urges each day. It seems obvious to me that we as men have a relatively good handle on controlling 95 percent of these impulses; it's that 5 percent that kicks us in the ass. Let's face it, impulsive sex is the riskiest of all for many reasons. Now, I'm not talking about a spontaneous moment of passion in the backseat of your car with your wife. I'm talking about those moments where we act without thinking things through, without considering the consequences and ramifications, or risk vs. reward, if you will. Impulsive sex leads to unwanted pregnancies, STDs, broken hearts, broken relationships, and broken homes. I think you would agree that no amount of momentary pleasure is worth any of that! Yet, every minute of every day some man, somewhere, is risking everything that he loves and that he has ever accomplished for a vagina. A president in Washington, D.C., a governor in New York, or a basketball coach in Kentucky—it doesn't matter who you are or what you do, we are all susceptible to these impulses. The fact is, some of us are able to control them and others aren't. In my case, it has become much easier to control them as I get older. I attribute this to three main reasons:

1. Maturity.
2. The older I get, the more it seems I have to risk by making stupid impulsive decisions.
3. It took me a while, and at least eight different girls threatening to commit suicide, to realize that being a "heartbreaker" wasn't as cool as it was made out to be.

Believe me, I'm not trying to say it's always easy. You could imagine some of the temptation I am faced with because of my position in the adult industry. Imagine being surrounded by young girls who are naked, willing, and looking to impress you. And now, because of the TV show, I get propositions with naked pictures from women all over the world. However, no matter how tempting the offer seems to be, I couldn't ever

Divorce will decrease a man's wealth by an average of 77 percent.

> "Bad marriages don't cause infidelity; infidelity causes bad marriages."—Frank Pittman

see risking the relationship I have or the respect of my son or the stability of the home I have worked so hard for over a vagina—or asshole, for that matter! For me, it is impossible to avoid all temptation. Having said that, I make a conscious effort to avoid as much of it as possible. Unless I'm being paid to appear, you won't find me in a bar, nightclub, or especially a strip club without Mirna at my side. These are what I call "sexually charged social environments"—places that, when I'm in a relationship, I avoid like I would being raped by Shaquille O'Neal as he sang "Tell me how my ass tastes!" If I want to spend time with the fellas, I'll invite them over to my place or head on over to theirs. When I do find myself in a situation that I feel is starting to move in a dangerous direction, I will either mention Mirna, allude to the relationship in some way, or remove myself from the situation entirely. That's just the way I choose to play it now based on my extensive knowledge of me!

So the next time you're faced with temptation, after you've taken a moment to think about the potential size of the waves of pleasure you're about to ride, take a longer moment to consider the damage you can potentially cause to yourself or others if those waves you're playing in churn themselves into a tsunami.

The bottom line is to try to understand why it is that you are cheating or have the desire to cheat. Why do I think this is so important? Because I believe that in almost any and every circumstance, cheating is a mistake that can lead to life-altering, if not devastating, consequences for all concerned. The reality is people cheat because they're immature, selfish, narcissistic, or drama junkies! You might be able to fool yourself into thinking it is a better option than splitting or divorcing, but it is really only a Band-Aid that will soon lose its adhesion due to your repeated attempts to wash away any evidence and guilt. Like following the trail marked "shortcut" only to find the path leads through a treacherous jungle inhabited by penis-eating cannibals, it is not the "easiest way" for sure! The wise, honorable man admits his mistakes, accepts the consequences associated with those mistakes—and moves on! Here are some other things you should know about cheating:

- Over 90 percent of men who cheat say they regret their actions.
- Over 61 percent of women were not able to forgive their spouses after the affair became known.
- 20 percent of women felt their love turn to hate within six months after they experienced betrayal.
- Only 25 percent of cheating men were willing to discuss their sexual desires with their partners/wives. Only 17 percent of these male cheaters knew anything of their partners'/wives' sexual needs.
- 69 percent of marriages fail after an affair has been admitted to or discovered.

For some men the reasons for cheating have nothing to do with emotions or feelings of neglect. These men simply do not have the strength to resist sexual temptation. They are not in control of their sexual impulses. In other words, they think with their schlongs, not their brains. This type of thinking can be very dangerous—not only because it makes a man susceptible to being unfaithful to a partner and irreparably damaging a relationship but because of the potential serious consequences not being in control of one's sexual impulses can have on the life of any man, no matter his relationship status. Becoming a perpetrator of date rape is one of the most common of these consequences. There is absolutely no excuse for this type of behavior—not the amount of alcohol you consumed, not the sexy outfit she was wearing, not the fact that she rubbed your cock while tonguing your ear—*no means no*, regardless of the activities that preceded it! There are no exceptions . . . well, maybe there is one exception, and I just so happen to have encountered that one exception. Her name was Sandra. I met her while playing blackjack at the Aladdin casino

"Ah, yes, divorce, from the Latin word meaning to rip out a man's genitals through his wallet."—Robin Williams

one night as I wound down from another day at the porn convention. She was my table waitress and was obviously flirting with me as I wasted my money. Sometime around one thirty A.M., Sandra slipped me a note:

> I get off in 30 min. If you want to get a drink, meet me out front at 2:15.

I was out front at 2:10 A.M. Sandra was a hot little blonde with big tits and toned legs. I was more than anxious to see where this might lead. Five minutes later, Sandra exited the hotel and told me to take a cab to the Peppermill Lounge. Apparently, hotel employees are not allowed to leave with patrons, so she would meet me there.

Inside the Peppermill, we found a secluded red velvet booth and settled in before ordering one of the house's special flaming fu-fu drinks for two. Three flaming fu-fus and a few long, wet kisses later we were hopping into a cab and heading to a cheap motel. Soon I was sitting on the bed and Sandra was doing a slow, seductive striptease out of her clothes. Next, she undressed me—starting with my shoes and working her way up, licking and kissing my body as she traveled north. We moved into some sixty-nine until she came all over my face while swallowing my cock at the same time. I flipped Sandra over and climbed on top as I slipped the tip of my swizzle stick into her wetness. Take a listen to what happened next:

Sandra: No.
Me: You want me to stop?
Sandra: No.
Me: Okay.

Now I started to slowly piston in and out of her coochie.

Sandra: No, no, no.
Me: You want me to stop?
Sandra: No!

My pace started to quicken.

Sandra: *No, no, no!*

Me: What's up with you? Do you want me to stop or what?

Sandra: Sorry, I can't help it. I like to fantasize that I'm being forced. Does it bother you?

Me: No, not as long as I know that you want to do this.

Sandra: Trust me, I want to do this! Your cock feels so good!

Actually, the whole submissive thing turned me on and I continued fucking her—now, getting the clue, in a more forceful, dominant manner. Sandra continued to say no throughout with an occasional *"Oh god"* thrown in. She wanted it hard and fast and I was more than willing to oblige. The phone rang but we ignored it. Soon she was screaming at the top of her lungs and the headboard was banging against the wall. The phone rang again and we ignored it again. "Spank me harder," she said, and I cracked that tushy a few good ones. Then suddenly, during an extremely loud round of no's from Sandra, two cops burst into our room with guns drawn. "Police, stop what you're doing! Get off the bed, get down on the floor facedown, and put your hands behind your head!"

Apparently, the person in the room next door heard Sandra screaming no, thought she was being raped, and called the front desk. The motel manager tried calling the room and knocking on the door before deciding it was a matter for the police. Of course after the police were able to talk to Sandra, they apologized and the motel comped us the room. Inconvenient,

"What's intriguing is that part of the new masculinity, or m-ness, is man's recognition that he needs a woman. This realization comes, ironically, during the Era of Female Independence, a time when man can be replaced by boy toys, female lovers, abstinence and even vibrators . . . Whereas men still need women, their traditional source of comfort and inspiration, women are increasingly less likely to feel the same about men and that's changing everything about the rules of the game."
—Marian Salzman

yes, but don't think that Sandra and I didn't pick up where we left off as soon as the coast was clear.

That is absolutely, positively the only exception to the "No means no" rule. Lucky me!

Don't Take a Good Woman for Granted

Recent studies suggest over 50 percent of married women feel neglected sexually. There are probably as many reasons for this as there are married women who don't think they're getting laid enough. The neglected woman, though, will generally attribute the lack of intimacy to one of two reasons: Her man is not attracted to her anymore or her man is having an affair. Either realization can be devastating to a woman. The truth is that it's probably a combination of quite a few things, like:

- The fact that a man's sex drive naturally decreases as he approaches his forties and a woman's sex drive naturally increases as she approaches her thirties.
- It's just not as exciting to have sex with the same woman for the 3,981st time.
- As men age, they naturally take on more responsibilities, which in turn can translate to more stress and less time for intimacy.

It really doesn't matter what the reason is if you have a good woman whom you love and care for! Now, you either stop procrastinating and start fucking her right and regular or she's gonna dump your ass! Don't think she won't, because she will not only kick you to the curb but she'll get into the best shape of her life and find herself a twenty-four-year-old stud with a MILF fetish to fuck her silly while you sit at home either wishing you had her back or trying to figure out how you're gonna get laid! That kind of irony is a sad reality for many men who were simply too damn lazy to fuck their wives enough. Because if you know your partner has an issue with the frequency of sex and you don't attempt to fix the problem, you're simply too fucking lazy! Remember, procrastination is much like masturbation—inevitably, you're only just fucking yourself! Unless you have a medical condition, you have no excuse. All those reasons or excuses you use just won't matter in the end . . . after she's gone! Now that I've made my point more than clear, let me give you a couple of tips to help you get over this hump . . .

Schedule Your Sex—I know you've been told that women like spontaneity, and they do! But at this point, I guarantee you that she couldn't give a shit about how, when, or where it happens, she just wants to get laid—period! Whether it's twice weekly or every day, you need to schedule the intimate time with her and stick to the schedule.

Remove the Television from Your Bedroom—I can hear some of you screaming, "But what about my late-night *SportsCenter* highlights?" I don't know what to tell you other than, it works! A survey by an Italian psychologist found that couples who did not have a TV in their bedroom had sex an average of seven times a month, compared to 1.5 times per month for couples with TVs. It seems that watching TV becomes a habit that translates into a lot less sex for many couples.

CHAPTER 11

Hairy Situations

Women appreciate a clean, well-groomed man. They are attracted to men who put an effort into their grooming. Now, I'm not suggesting you become a full-fledged metrosexual, I'm just suggesting you become conscious of your appearance and hygiene, especially the following:

Skin—While rough skin on a man might indicate a certain amount of machismo, it doesn't feel nearly as good to a woman as smooth skin does. This is just a matter of finding a good body lotion to apply to yourself after showering and good hand/face lotions to apply as needed.

Lips—Women hate kissing a pair of chapped lips. Is it so hard to carry a lip balm around with you, especially during wintertime, when your lips are more likely to get chapped?

Nails—I'm talking about both your finger- and toenails. Women are especially quick to notice hands and feet. Aside from the aesthetic benefits of taking care of your fingernails, there is an additional sexual benefit—sharp, uneven fingernails can cause damage to a woman's pussy and/or ass. Nothing will kill a woman's mood quicker than having her pussy torn to shreds during foreplay! Keep those nails clean and trimmed.

Ears—No woman wants to stick her tongue in your ear and pull it out covered in wax. Yes, women love candles but not when they're growing out of your ears. Use Q-tips after every shower. Pluck your ear hairs if you got 'em.

Nose—If you look like you have a pair of furry caterpillars stuffed up your nostrils, trim those fuckers. They even make electric nose-hair trimmers for those of you who aren't good with a pair of tweezers.

Back—If it looks like you're still wearing a wool sweater after you just removed your wool sweater, you might want to consider one of the methods of hair removal I discuss below.

Ass—Personally, I shave mine. Although, sometimes Mirna will shave it for me. In either case it's done in the shower with a good sharp razor (Mach3 or double-edged) and plenty of moisturizing shaving cream. If I'm doing it myself, I simply bend over and shave it by using my free hand to spread my cheeks. I shave it from crack out and try to avoid passing over the same area numerous times. This will help keep razor burn or irritation to a minimum.

Whether you decide to shave your ass or have your partner shave it is really more of a matter of personal preference than anything; however, keeping your ass meticulously clean is an absolute must! Going down on a guy with a stinky ass hasn't made any of the turn-on lists I've seen attributed to women. I keep a box of baby wipes by every toilet in our house. After using a little toilet paper first, I always finish the job with a baby wipe to make sure my asshole is sparkling clean. I also make sure to always wipe my ass from front to back—starting from where my ass crack meets my taint and moving away from my balls. I always make sure to give my ass a quick once-over before I'm going to do the dirty deed. If I don't

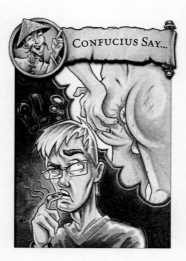

Man who scratch ass should not bite fingernails

have a baby wipe handy, I'll lean my ass over the sink and splash water on it and then use toilet paper to dry myself and check for cleanliness. Go ahead and say it . . . "He's anal about his anus." Yeah, could it be due to my enjoyment of having my salad tossed? I expect my partner's to be spic and span for sex and see no reason why she shouldn't expect the same of me! And by the way, if you're into having your salad tossed or the occasional prostate massage, you'll need to even take things a step further—like showering before sex and using a finger along with "no tears" shampoo to clean your ass. Some men prefer enemas before sex as opposed to the finger routine, which is fine as long as you don't drink the enema! (See chapter 22.)

Cock and Balls—Obviously, you want to keep your twig and berries clean! This is especially important to remember for those of you with uncut cocks. The other issue here is shaving. Many men today are trimming their pubes—some at the request of a woman, others because they know that it makes their dicks look bigger. It really doesn't matter why, because studies show women prefer to feel a smooth cock and balls; sounds like a win-win proposition to me. Here are a few things to remember when shaving your cock and balls:

1. Use a clean, sharp razor each time.
2. Always shave in the shower or immediately after you shower. It is best to shave when the hair is wet.
3. Always shave in the direction of the hair growth.
4. Avoid passing the razor over the same area repeatedly.
5. When shaving your balls, use your free hand to stretch the skin tightly.
6. When shaving your cock or your balls, go slowly and for god's sake be fucking careful!

The only drawbacks to shaving are the potential loss of blood and the fact that you have to do it quite regularly in order to stay smooth and avoid irritating your partner—literally. Of course, nowadays shaving isn't your only hair-removal option. Many men, not just metrosexuals, are using both laser and waxing removal methods.

Laser Hair Removal—Laser hair removal works by targeting melanin (the dark pigment that gives hair its color). As the laser's light is absorbed by the melanin, the resulting heat kills the surrounding hair follicles. Lasers can be used to remove hair from your face, legs, back, chest, underarms, ass, and genitals. Each area that you target will need an initial six to eight laser treatments spaced six to ten weeks apart. Your genetics will determine how often you will need follow-up treatments. This method is certainly more expensive than both shaving and waxing, with treatments ranging between $100 and $850 in the US, but will also keep you smooth for a much longer period of time. There is a minimal amount of pain involved as the laser will produce a slight burning sensation.

Waxing—Waxing will keep the hair away longer than shaving but not as long as laser removal. It is without a doubt the most painful of the three options. Let's face it, your hair is literally being ripped out of your skin. Despite the pain factor, genital waxing is becoming popular among men, as demonstrated by the acknowledgments from both P. Diddy and Jay-Z that they are waxees. Some waxing salons have even renamed the traditional bikini and Brazilian (front, rear, and every-thing in between) waxing services normally targeted to women as the "mankini" and "manzilian." Waxing is also a very effective method of hair removal for your face, legs, back, chest, underarms, ass, and geni-tals. It is moderately expensive, with treatments ranging between $30 and $60 per area.

Take a look at my pre-sex hygiene checklist. When possible, I try to always do these things right before I am going to have sex:

- ☐ Make sure my cock, balls, ass, taint, and everywhere in between is clean. Whether I do this in the shower or with baby wipes, it really doesn't matter. Hell, if I have no other options, I'll sit my ass on the sink and splash water on myself—a poor man's bidet, if you will.
- ☐ Clean my ears.
- ☐ Blow my nose. I do this for two reasons: to make sure I don't have boogers hanging out and to clear my breathing passages. A man can suffocate himself when eating pussy with a stuffed-up nose!

There are medical conditions that can result in the growth of pubic hair on boys and girls as early as eighteen months old.

☐ Check my nails for sharp edges. If I find some, I'll file them down quickly or bite them off if I have to.

☐ Make sure my hands, feet, and toes are clean. You never know when you might run into a woman who loves to do this:

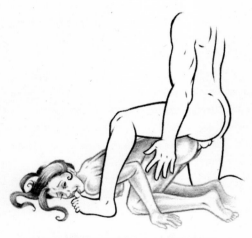

"That's right, suck those toes while I bury my cock in your hot pussy!"

☐ Apply deodorant.

☐ Brush my teeth or gargle with mouthwash.

☐ Ready to rock her world.

Only 18 percent of men remove hair from their privates, compared to 95 percent of women.

BOOK II
ABOUT HER

CHAPTER 12

The Mating Game

There aren't a lot of subjects you could get a group of women to agree on, but when it comes to pickup lines there's a strong consensus. Most women will tell you they find pickup lines cheesy and an insult to their intelligence. They will tell you that they much prefer a straightforward approach—"Hi, I'm Adam, can I buy you a drink?" They will tell you that they want a guy's confidence to be evident. They will tell you that they want to be approached when they're with a group of other women and appreciate a guy's "courage" when he does so. They will tell you that they want the guy to look directly in their eyes when he speaks (never underestimate the power of direct eye contact in all types of social and business settings).

This is the way I do it. I stopped resorting to gimmicks to meet women long ago. That's not to say that all pickup lines won't work or that I don't think that there are some effective strategies for meeting women. I also understand that some of you guys just feel more comfortable using a stale line. In my opinion, these tactics are like a shield that protects you from letting a girl see your weaknesses. But the problem is that women see your shield for what it is.

Whether you're using lines or a more honest approach, meeting women is a numbers game. The more you approach, the more chances you have of meeting someone you like and who likes you. Now, that last part of that last sentence is key! Everything I've written prior to this is based on the assumption you're looking to meet someone who you could have a "real" relationship with. If it's a one-night stand you're looking for, the use of gimmick lines can be highly effective. Just be aware of the

"I think men talk to women so they can sleep with them and women sleep with men so they can talk to them."
—Jay McInerny

reasons why they work. First, there is only a certain percentage of women who are even open to the idea of having a one-night stand. These women will tend to have self-esteem issues. Second, alcohol and/or drugs will usually play a part in those women's decision-making process. Finally, one last thing to consider: Maybe these women are receptive to the gimmicks because they have an alternative agenda, like getting pregnant and milking you for money for the next eighteen years of your life.

Never forget, meeting women is a very competitive game. Despite the fact that population statistics say there are more women in this world than men, it is a rare occasion to be at a party or nightclub where the men are outnumbered by the women. The same way Fortune 500 companies compete for market share and attempt to make their brands stand out above the rest, men are faced with the same challenges when attempting to meet women. Whether we like it or not, women will always be judging us, even before they meet us, with respect to the way we dress, our personal grooming and hygiene standards, the state of our physiques, and the very first words that come out of our mouths. Speaking of physiques, let me take a moment to make suggestions . . .

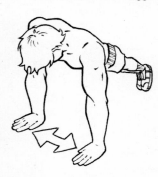

Standard push-up position

If you were limited to doing one exercise for the rest of your life, push-ups would be the call. It is the best single exercise because it engages the most major muscle groups, including the pectorals (chest), deltoids (shoulders), latismus (back), and triceps (back of arm), plus they can be done at any time, anywhere—with no special equipment needed. On top of all that, push-ups will pump you up faster than Dr. 90210 pumps up a flat-chested girl—every macho action star in Hollywood does a few sets immediately before stepping in front of the camera! Once you become accustomed to doing the standard push-up, there is a host of variations you could add to increase difficulty or change up the focus of the exercise.

Feet Up—Take the standard push-up position with your palms flat on the floor but place your feet on a low chair or couch. This will essentially increase the amount of work you have to do to get your chest back up off the floor, increasing both the difficulty and effectiveness of the exercise.

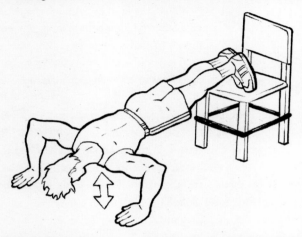

Varying Hand Positions—The standard push-up position calls for you to place your hands shoulder-width apart. By placing your hands farther apart, you will be adding extra stress to your delts, lats, and outer pecs. By placing your hands closer together, you will be placing the extra workload on the center of your chest as well as your triceps. These techniques should be especially helpful for those of you looking to improve your upper-body symmetry.

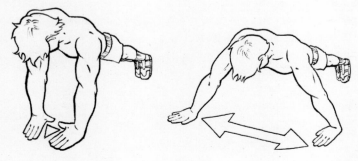

Plyometrics—These are types of exercises or variations on exercises that are meant to add the component of building "explosive strength and speed." In the case of push-ups, the variation calls for you to assume the standard 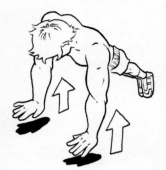 position, lowering your chest to the ground as normal. The plyometric component is achieved as you push yourself back up with enough force to actually lift your upper body, hands and all, entirely off the floor as your feet remain stationary. At first you'll only be able to get your hands an inch or two off the floor, if at all. But with practice, you'll find you'll actually be able to clap your hands in between each push-up.

Now let's get back on topic. As I was saying, our dress, hygiene, physical fitness, and verbal skills are all part of that most important "first impression" that we all have heard so much about. While all the factors mentioned above are important, those first words—and the manner in which you deliver them—are likely to be the deciding factor, unless, of course, your dazzling good looks have dazzled her enough that she doesn't care what comes out of your mouth. Whether I like it or not, there are some guys that do seem to have success based solely on their physical appearance. I am certainly not suggesting that you get obsessive over your appearance, as this will suggest a lack of self-confidence to many women. Sure, you may have a beer belly or a big nose or a bald head, but I'm here to tell you that there are women out there who find each of those so-called physical flaws to be physical assets. Yet some of us men will go to extreme lengths to fix or hide them instead of understanding there really is no such thing as physical perfection. As a younger man, I was one of these guys. I wore a hat every day of tenth grade to cover my ugly curly hair and avoided wearing shorts whenever possible into my midtwenties in order to hide my flamingo legs. It took a while for me to finally realize that what

"If you can't dazzle them with brilliance, baffle them with bull."
—W. C. Fields

"A man can be short and dumpy and getting bald but if he has fire, women will like him."—Mae West

I said to a woman and how I said it was so much more important than if I was having a bad hair day or not! Yes, first physical impressions and your overall appearance are important, but they are certainly not things to become obsessive over.

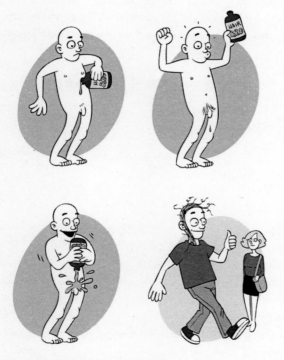

There are two types of gimmicks that men use to meet women: the conversational opener and the pickup line. If I had to choose, I would recommend the use of conversational openers because they give you the opportunity to engage her in a somewhat substantial conversation right off the bat, as opposed to casting a cheese-baited hook and seeing if she bites. Now, I could say that every one of the "gimmicks" I'm about to give you will work every time, but that would be an outright lie. I couldn't say it because I know the reaction of any particular woman is dependent upon any number of uncontrollable factors. Who's delivering the line, how the line is delivered, and to whom the line is being delivered will all play deciding roles. As I've said time and again, every woman is different to some degree or another. Some women won't give you the time of day if they even catch a whiff of "game." You need to understand that much of your success, or lack thereof, will be dependent on your ability to assess each individual set of circumstances—where you happen to be at the time of your approach and whom you happen to be approaching. Having said all that, with disclaimers firmly in place and without further ado, here are some of the best strategies to meet women I've ever come across.

Conversational Opener #1

The Suit Opener

Approaching a female or a group of females, you say, "Could you help me? We need a female's opinion."

> **Female(s):** Yes, sure, etc.
>
> **You:** My buddy has a problem. He owns two suits. One he has worn to church [or temple] every Sunday for the last three years and one is a beautiful Armani suit that he never wears because he never goes anywhere nice enough. The problem is his ex-girlfriend bought him the Armani suit and he wants to wear it to a wedding he's taking his current girlfriend to. His current girlfriend said she's not going if he wears it. What do you think he should do?

At this point she is fully engaged in your "problem" and she has already made a few observations about you: You're a good friend trying to help out a buddy with a problem. You might have some fashion sense, as you clearly recognize the Armani brand as high-end. You're probably a nice guy because you have churchgoing friends.

Conversational Opener #2

The Puppy Opener

Approaching a female or a group of females, you say, "I'm wondering if you ladies could help me with something."

> **Female(s):** How can we help?
>
> **You:** I was in a long-term relationship that ended about six months ago. We got a puppy when we moved in together and the dog became an issue when we were splitting up. So I let her take the dog instead of having to go to court over it. That was six months ago and now I've decided to get another puppy. My buddies are trying to tell me that women judge men by the type of dog they own. I want to get a Chihuahua and they're saying some women will assume I'm gay because of it.

Now she's fully engaged, and here are some of the observations she has already made about you: You're single. You're an animal lover. You're not gay.

I will warn you that using this opener could lead to some backstory follow-up questions that you'd better be prepared for, like "Why did you break up?" "How long were you living together?" "What kind of dog was it?" and "What was its name?"

Conversational Opener #3

The Book Opener

Approaching a female in a bookstore, you say, "I was wondering if you could give me some advice on something."

> **Female:** What do you need?
>
> **You:** I have a cousin turning eighteen and I wanted to give her a

"Women speak two languages—one of which is verbal."
—Unknown

book that would really help her understand what young women today face out there in the real world. Would you happen to have any suggestions for me?

Now she's fully engaged, and here are some of the observations she has already made about you: You're family oriented. You're compassionate toward others. You're well-read. You're thoughtful. You're intelligent.

Conversational Opener #4

The Gym Opener

Approaching a female at a gym, you say, "Can I get your opinion on something really quick?"

Female: Sure.

You: My buddy over there joined this gym over two years ago. He joined with his girlfriend but they broke up nine months ago. Now my buddy is in a new relationship and his current girlfriend wants him to stop working out here because his ex-girlfriend is still a member. I told him I think his girlfriend is being a bit immature but I'm wondering what your thoughts are on it.

Now she's fully engaged, and here are some of the observations she has made about you: You're a concerned friend. You take care of your body. You have a mature outlook.

Conversational Opener #5

The Can Opener
(My All-Time Favorite)

Approaching a female or a group of females, you say, "Can I bother you for a little advice?"

Female(s): What's the problem?

You: My buddy over there was thrown out of his house by his fiancée three days ago. It was their two-year anniversary and he gave her a beautiful diamond tennis bracelet and took her to a fantastic restaurant, but he also asked her if they could have anal sex together. She freaked out, accused him of being a closet homosexual, and threw him out of the house. Now she wants him to come home but never mention anal sex again! He's asking me for advice, and I have no idea what to tell him to do.

Now she's fully engaged, and here are some of the observations she has made about you: You're a concerned friend. You're liberal-minded. You know something about jewelry. You're not gay.

I say this one's my all-time favorite because it not only accomplishes the same as the other openers but also garners an opinion on anal sex. Which, to an anal freak such as myself, can be very helpful!

I would encourage you to get creative devising your own personal conversational openers. You won't deliver any opener more confidently than one you've devised yourself. However, no matter where you get your opener, you always must keep this in mind: Using a conversational opener is a method of starting a conversation with a woman, plain and simple. This conversation, which has nothing to do with your true intentions, is solely a tool you are using to get a woman to feel comfortable enough with you to accept an invitation for a drink, dinner, or a trip back to your pad.

Once you exceed the conversational limits of your opener you will need to be prepared to close her. Here are examples of some effective closing lines:

- "Wow, you should be writing an advice column. Can I show you my appreciation with a drink?"
- "I really appreciate you taking the time to hear me out and I think your advice is right on! Would you like to join me at my table for a drink?"
- "I really enjoyed our conversation! Can I take you to dinner so we can continue it?"
- "I really like the way you think! Is there any way we can get together later so I can learn more about you?"

Pickup Lines

I will break these down into two categories for you: blunt-force lines and soft and smooth lines.

Examples of Blunt-Force Lines

- Once you've made eye contact with her, beckon her over to you using the "come hither" motion with your index finger. When she comes over to see what you want, you tell her, "Oh, I don't want anything . . . I just wanted to see if I could make you come with this finger."
- "Nice shoes; wanna fuck?"
- "Would you rather hook up with a 'bad boy' who has a really big dick but is a selfish lover or a nice guy who has an average-size dick but is a fantastic lover?" (This one could be used as an opener if you develop it more.)
- Dip your finger in a glass of water, then touch her thigh and say, "Let's go back to my place and get you out of these wet clothes!"

- "Are you looking for Mr. Right or Mr. Right Now?"
- "That outfit looks incredible on you, but I think it would look even better lying on the floor next to my bed!"

Blunt-force lines like these will either get you slapped or get you laid. Either way I caution you to use them with discretion!

Examples of Soft and Smooth Lines

- "Do you believe in love at first sight? If not, I'll walk by again."
- "Can I ask your opinion on something? Do these pants make my ass look fat?"
- "I couldn't help noticing you and I'm hoping you're the kind of woman to know the difference between a pickup line and a sincere compliment. You look fantastic in that outfit! My name's _____."
- Ask if you can tell her a story. Then pick up her hand and draw an imaginary line across it and then place an imaginary dot on one side of the line. Tell her the dot is a little puppy and the line is a busy highway. The puppy has to get across the highway. Then tell her she has three chances to guess how the puppy could cross the road. No matter what she guesses, you'll say no. When she's exhausted her three available choices, she'll ask for the correct answer, at which time you'll respond, "I have no idea, I just wanted to hold your hand."
- "I've been killing myself trying to figure out who it is you remind me of and it just came to me. You look exactly like my next girlfriend."
- "My friend just bet me fifty dollars that I couldn't strike up a conversation with the prettiest girl at the club. If you talk with me for a minute, drinks are on me."

Soft and smooth lines like these will generally be received with a smile because of their inoffensive wording. At the very worst, you'll get a polite "Buzz off!"

"All women think they're ugly, even pretty women. A man who understands this could fuck more women than Don Giovanni. They all think their cunts are ugly. They all find fault with their figures. Even models and actresses, even women you think are so beautiful that they have nothing to worry about do worry all the time."—Erica Jong

Best Places to Meet Women

1. **Coffee Shops**—Quickly catching up to bars and nightclubs as the place to meet people, without the loud music and drooling drunks. Coffee shops offer a relaxed atmosphere that is conducive to striking up conversations. The interiors and amenities (free Wi-Fi) encourage people to spend extended periods in these shops, which should give you the time to get your shit together and approach her with a proper opener. Whether you prefer to frequent coffee shops, bars, or restaurants, I do want to take a moment to discuss tipping etiquette. If I get exceptional service, I believe in tipping appropriately. That could mean a 25 to 30 percent tip, but it will also translate into great service every time I'm at that establishment. I will always tip between 15 and 20 percent on most other occasions. In general, 15 percent is considered to be the "polite standard" here in the United States; however, these standards do change from country to country. If you do happen to have a few favorite spots you like to take dates to, I would recommend tipping at a higher scale at these establishments as it's always nice to be treated well and with respect by the staff—plus this will not go unnoticed by your date!

2. **Yoga Classes**—A great place to meet women for a couple of reasons. First, it presents you with the opportunity for continuous and regular run-ins with her. Second, it establishes right off the bat that you both have at least one thing in common, plus it provides you with a topic for conversation that you already know she's interested in—whether it be physical fitness in general or yoga specifically. Finally, you'll have

plenty of time to check out each other's bodies—which can be an advantage or disadvantage to you depending upon the shape you're in!

3. **Fitness Boot Camps**—For the exact same reasons as above.

4. **Music Stores**—Music stores are great places to meet women because they are generally in browsing mode when shopping for music, which gives you time to get your game plan straight before you make your play. Also, listening to music will likely put the woman in a good mood, making her more receptive to a well-thought-out approach. The conversational potential is plentiful and should be obvious to you by now! However, just in case you opened the book up to this page and started reading, I'll give you a few ideas:

- "Have you heard this album? I've only heard the single and I'm not sure if I want to buy the whole album."
- "I'm looking for a present for my fourteen-year-old cousin. Could you recommend some groups she may be into?"

5. **Sports Bars**—Assuming that you're a sports fan, what could be better than meeting a woman you're attracted to and can talk about the game with? Here the conversation should flow as readily as the alcohol, with a variety of topics to be explored.

6. **Dog Parks**—Women who love animals are attracted to men who love animals—plain and simple! Dog parks provide great opportunities for easy, no-pressure conversational openers:

- "What's your dog's name?"
- "How old is your dog?"
- "Do you know of any other dog parks in the area?"
- "Do you know of a good groomer?"
- "Can you recommend a good vet?"

In my opinion, those are the best places to meet women. Now I want to tell you about one of the worst. For some reason, many men think strip clubs are good places to meet women, which is true if you're looking for a woman to drain your wallet instead of your balls. If you are getting your balls drained at a strip club I can guarantee you're paying extra for the service and yours aren't the only balls being drained by that stripper. Like Vegas casinos, strip clubs are designed to relieve you of your money, and the women who work there are highly trained seductresses used to speed the process along. Most strippers will tell you the key to their success, aside from their stunning good looks or perfect tits, is their ability to make a man (customer) feel special—make a man feel that she has a genuine interest in him. And 99 percent of the time, she does have a genuine interest . . . in his money only. Strippers are basically commissioned sales executives who happen to remove their clothes as part of their job. They all have the common goal of establishing a stable of regulars—lonely guys who spend lots of money and visit the club regularly. Most will say anything and some will do even more than that to establish and maintain a relationship with these men, much like a con artist milking an easy mark. Many strippers don't even like men, and most of the rest have an unemployed musician with a fondness for crystal meth waiting for them in the parking lot. Take it from a guy who's had many strippers sit upon his lap: Strip clubs are not good places to meet women!

Avoid Turning Women Off

Men make many mistakes with women during the introductory "getting to know you" phase. Unfortunately, this is the most crucial phase, as it is the time she is going to be making a majority of her assumptions about the man pursuing her. Actually, now that I think about it, using the word "mistakes" here is a cop-out—these are really behavioral patterns, as men are prone to repeat them over and over. Here is a list of the most common behavioral patterns that will turn women off quickly:

Eager Beaver Syndrome—Women don't want things made too easy for them. They enjoy a bit of mystery and the thrill of the chase. They love the gamesmanship aspect of relationships. Not only do you have to be willing to play the game, but you've got to establish your own set of rules. For our purposes, we can call them a list of behavioral guidelines that you set for yourself and follow.

A. Don't call her for a minimum of twenty-four hours after getting her phone number.

B. Don't answer the phone every time she calls. Even if you are available, let it go to voice mail to make her wonder what you might be doing.

C. Hold back some details—don't reveal your entire schedule to her. Being vague about your activities and whereabouts adds mystery and will pique her interest. For instance . . .

Girl: What did you do last night?
You: Went out with some friends and had a few drinks.
Girl: A guys' night out?
You: You could say that.

D. If you call her and she does not return your call, wait one week and try again. If she does not return that call, move on, she's not interested!

Nice Guy Syndrome—Being too nice can turn a woman off faster than I ejaculated during my first sexual experience! It's also a way of giving up your power before you've even gotten into a relationship. You don't have to agree with everything she says, do everything she asks, or laugh at all her jokes—especially if they're not funny!

Master Debater Syndrome—You can't convince a woman to like you no matter how compelling an argument you think you can make. When you find yourself resorting to having to say things like "But didn't we have great sex?" "I will treat you so much better than him!" "What about all those things you said?" or "What about all the plans we made together?" forget about it, because it's time to move on and save yourself frustration and heartache! Continue this pattern and you will become a "Master Bater"!

Can't Buy Me Love Syndrome—I'd like to say that you can't buy a woman's love, but we all know that's not true. That being said, is it something you really want to do? The guys who have to resort to this tactic will eventually have to face the stark reality that there is always another man out there with more money than them.

Heart on Sleeve Syndrome—I don't care if you feel like your heart's gonna explode every time you see her or if you've "never felt this way before" after a first date—you just can't tell her these types of things early in the relationship. This type of talk ends any illusion of a chase she might have had and removes all scent of mystery from you. If you feel the uncontrollable need to express yourself, write it down in letters. Later, you can decide whether you want to destroy them or give them to her as a present on your first wedding anniversary.

While making every effort to avoid turning women off is a good thing, allowing yourself to become pussy-whipped is not. You need to realize that just by reading this book you are adding to your value as a man, and if you start implementing the suggestions made here, you will become an even rarer commodity. A man should never be willing to sacrifice his pride or integrity for the sake of getting laid. There is no pussy worth sacrificing your pride and integrity for. Remember, for every woman you find yourself attracted to, there is a man tired of both her and her vagina. A man like you should never feel grateful to be spending time with a dynamite woman—appreciative yes, grateful no. Consider the fact that most men don't have a clue as to how women's bodies work and couldn't give a damn either! Consider the fact that only 29 percent of women report they have regular orgasms during sex. Consider the fact that there are more women in the world than men in general. Consider all these things the next time you think about swallowing your pride for the sake of getting laid.

Online Dating

The Internet has changed the game of dating completely. Whereas most people were restricted to playing locally on their home fields, nowadays there's no such thing as out-of-bounds. I used to consider a girl "geographically undesirable" if she lived more than a tank of gas away. Now I can share as much intimate, face-to-face time with a woman in Siberia as I could with someone who lived down the street if I chose. I know couples who met in person for the very first time within days of getting married. Any of you familiar with my television show will remember that I have had my own interesting experiences with online dating. While I didn't make a love connection myself, I do think it is something anyone looking for that special someone should consider, if for no other reason than the sheer convenience of being able to browse through unlimited profiles of single women. Of course, this convenience comes with a price. Dating sites will charge some sort of membership fee, and oh, by the way, the competition online is fierce. Lucky for you, you'll have the advantage if you pay attention to the following words.

The first task you face is choosing a site. To save you some time and energy, I have put together a list of the twelve online dating sites that I would check out if I were single today:

Match.com
Chemistry.com
Singlesnet.com
Jdate.com (Jewish) (US only)
Bigchurch.com (Christian)
Date.com
Perfectmatch.com
Blacksingles.com (black) (US only)
Amigos.com (Latin)
Amor.com (Latin)
Plentyoffish.com (no fees)
Lavalife.com (US, Canada and Australia only)

Once you've chosen the site, your next step will be your most important one—creating your dating profile. Half-ass it on your profile, and you might as well flush your money down the toilet. Your profile is your all-important first impression online. It is your sell sheet, catalog, pitch brochure—whatever you prefer to call it. You'll need to step outside

It is estimated that over twenty-five million Americans visit at least one online dating site per month. There will be over 150,000 marriages in 2009 that occur as a result of online dating.

"Computer dating is fine . . . if you're a computer."
—Rita Mae Brown

yourself and perceive "you" as a product, like those products you see on TV that are sold by the millions by those slick, fast-talking salesman. As if you were selling ShamWows or the Bowflex, you must sell yourself. Here are some tips that will help you create a great dating profile:

Choose a Distinctive Username—This is the "nickname" you will be asked to choose. It should be memorable, creative, and a reflection of you. For example, "Snatchsniffer," "DesperateinDetroit," or "SuicidalinSeattle" just ain't gonna cut the mustard.

Write Creative, Humorous Headlines—Leave the sentiment for the ladies and avoid negativity all together. Make her smile or laugh while reading your profile and you've got her attention. When I was on Jdate, I would alternate my headline between "Jew talking to me?" and "I made over $18,000 at my bar mitzvah!" Changing your headline up every so often will keep your profile fresh and let women know you're engaged in the process.

Post Two Photos Minimum—These should be good photos but not necessarily the best photos you've ever taken in your life. It is more important that they be recent and indicative of your personal spirit, whether they show you at a party with friends, jumping off a cliff in Mexico, or at the base of a pyramid in Egypt. These types of photos are more likely to heighten a woman's interest, as opposed to a shot of you sitting on a floral-print couch. I would also recommend you include a picture you have with a pet(s), if that applies to you. Women with a love for animals will award you bonus points for sharing their affection.

Focus on Your Unique Qualities—"I love working out and watching wrestling" is most likely going to be the last thing a woman wants to read. And it will be if you include a line like that in your profile, as most women will immediately lose interest and move on to the next very convenient profile with the push of a button. Come on, there's got to be more to you

"Bisexuality immediately doubles your chances for a date on Saturday night."—Woody Allen

than that. Do you excel at a particular sport or have any unusual skill sets? Perhaps you won a yodeling contest while vacationing in Switzerland or maybe you can play the banjo while standing on your head. If I spoke another language, held the world record for eating matzo balls, grew award-winning cucumbers, climbed Mount Everest, worked on Obama's election campaign, or could touch my eyelids with my tongue, you can be sure I would include it in my profile.

Be Specific—Especially when you get to the part about what you're looking for in a woman. Doing this will serve as a filter to help you avoid wasting time with women who don't meet your criteria.

Be Honest—The last thing you want to do is start a relationship off dishonestly. If you lie about your age, weight, or height, or post a photo of yourself that's ten years old, it will inevitably catch up to you and take a bite out of your ass.

Chek Ur Grammer n Speling—And stay away from those stupid text abbreviations. You don't want to come across looking like an uneducated moron, do you?

Now that you have put together a profile that doesn't suck, it's time to take the field. Remember, though, the rules of the game are slightly different in the virtual world. Here are a few things to keep in mind:

Be Aware—Just because you're being honest doesn't mean everyone else is. Don't be afraid to ask direct questions, like "Is that a recent picture?" or "Is

"Sex appeal is fifty percent what you've got and fifty percent what people think you've got."—Sophia Loren

> "If you tell the truth you don't have to remember anything."
> —Mark Twain

that your real age?" or "Do you have children?" Any women with online dating experience will understand why you may be a tad suspicious.

Be Open-Minded—Try not to forget that not everyone is photogenic. There are some people who just don't take good photos and vice versa. Try not to base your interest solely on the pictures in a profile.

Stay Engaged—Get into the habit of checking your account daily if possible and reply promptly (within twenty-four hours) when someone expresses interest.

Don't Be Pushy—Being direct is different from being pushy. Try not to immediately barrage a woman with a hailstorm of personal questions. Let the conversation progress naturally. Pushing for immediate phone contact or an in-person meeting will turn most women off faster than homeless man toes. Let her dictate the pace of such things.

Assuming you've been paying attention, you will eventually get to the first phone call. Here are some tips to make it go as smoothly as possible:

What to Talk About—Aside from the obvious, you should be able to glean plenty of potential topics of conversation from her profile. Generally, they will include areas of likes and dislikes, or turn-ons and turnoffs, or "favorite" lists, etc. Look for topics that you share a common interest in or anything that stands out to you, for that matter. There's nothing wrong with preparing some notes on potential topics of conversation to use during that first call. You could take it a step further and have a joke or two at the ready. For instance, if I noticed that she owned a cat, I might look for an opportunity to say something like this:

> Do you know the difference between dogs and cats?
> Dogs come when you call them, while cats take a message and get
>   back to you later.

If you get this far and still want to meet the chick, I'd like to toss out the following for you to consider:

Prepare yourself for the first meeting just as you did for the first phone call—just don't bring the notes with you or write them on the palm of your hand. If you see any red flags or have an uneasy feeling about a face-to-face, you could always suggest an introductory videoconference online to break the ice. When you are ready to discuss your first face-to-face, be prepared with a variety of suggestions for your first meeting. Here is a list of places to go/things to do that I would suggest:

ACTIVITY	COMMENT
Coffee Lunch	Coffee or lunch as opposed to dinner—either will offer a more casual atmosphere while providing an easier escape if necessary.
Take a Walk	Whether it be on the beach, through her neighborhood, or a short hike, it's the face time and opportunity to talk that's important here.
Mini-Golf Catch Frisbee Batting cages Smashball Tennis Shoot hoops	If she has indicated she's athletic, all of these activities are great opportunities for easy communication. Plus, it's a chance for you to impress her with your skills.

Conversely to the above, I would suggest you avoid the following activities for that first meeting: dinner, movies, bars, and nightclubs.

Finally, if all goes well that first rendezvous, send her an e-mail later that evening along the lines of the following:

Just wanted to let you know what a nice time I had with you tonight!
Sweet dreams

Her response should say it all. She will either reply promptly expressing a similar sentiment or, even better, suggest that you get together again—or she will wait a few days before sending a "Dear John"–type reply or not reply altogether. In any case, you will have a good idea of where you stand with her.

Female Body Language

As I mentioned before, being a good listener is a key to understanding women. However, you can also gain valuable insight about how a woman is feeling by being able to read her body language. This can be especially helpful during those first conversations you have with women at bars or clubs before you have decided to attempt to close the deal or not. By being able to read her body language, you will have a good idea if she has any interest in getting to know you better before you open yourself up to potential rejection. Now, take a look at the chart below to get a better understanding of what I'm talking about.

Female Body Language Decoder Chart

ACTION	MEANING	
	SHE'S INTERESTED	SHE'S NOT INTERESTED
Touches You During Conversation	X	
Leans in toward You	X	
Twirls Hair with Finger	X	
Tosses Hair to Reveal Neck	X	
Legs or Shoulders Pointed at You	X	
Applies Lip Gloss in Front of You	X	
Uses Fingers to Play with Her Ears or Lips	X	
Makes Direct Eye Contact	X	
Dangles One Shoe with Foot While Sitting Cross-Legged	X	
Leans Away from You		X
Crosses Arms		X
Doesn't Make Direct Sustained Eye Contact		X
Throws Drink at You		X
Kicks You in Balls		X

Male Body Language

Reading body language isn't only a skill that men can practice. Women are doing it as well—whether they realize it or not. Some are consciously analyzing your movements, while others are subconsciously taking note—but they're all doing it, which makes it essential for you to become aware of your own body language and what it is saying to women. Here is a male body language decoder chart that will make things clearer for you . . .

Male Body Language Decoder Chart

ACTION	WHAT IT PROJECTS
Standing tall and straight	You're a self-confident man.
Holding eye contact until she drops	Not only are you self-confident but you're interested in her. If you look away before she does, you have put yourself in an inferior position.
Fidgety hands/quick movements	You're self-conscious with low self-esteem—why else would you be so nervous?
Crossing your arms	This is a defensive stance and will make women feel that they should stay away from you.
Leaning in close/invading her personal space	Getting too close too soon can be a major turnoff. It screams that you are only interested in sex with her.
Leading with your head while you walk	This makes you look slightly hunched and gives off the impression that you're a guy with low self-esteem who thinks too much.
Leading with your belly while you walk	This will give the impression that you're a weaker individual who is guided by his emotions and appetite.
Leading with your pelvis while you walk	You're a man of high self-esteem with sexual confidence and experience.
Drooling	You're a loser.
Rubbing your crotch while staring at her	You're a pervert.

Look, none of what you just read guarantees you won't be rejected. Dealing with rejection is a necessary evil when playing the mating game. Dwelling on the rejection or trying to make sense of it will only take time away from what you should truly be concerned with: finding your next target. I know that these words won't be enough to keep some of you from obsessing over your next rejection, so I thought the following would help make things clearer for you:

Interpreting the Top Eight Reasons Women Reject Men

WHAT SHE SAYS	WHAT SHE MEANS
"I've got a boyfriend."	I'd rather watch my cat cough up hairballs than go out with you.
"It's not you, it's me."	It's you!
"My life is too complicated right now."	I know ten other guys I'd rather spend my time with.
"I think of you more like a brother."	I don't date immature assholes.
"I think the difference in our ages would get in the way."	I don't screw old men.
"I'm concentrating on my career."	I'd rather tar roofs in Arizona during the middle of summer than waste my time with you.
"We're better off as friends."	I need a male companion to offer me his perspective after I give him all the juicy details of my love life.
"I'm celibate."	I don't fuck guys who look like you.

The truth of the matter is, who gives a damn why she rejected you—it doesn't matter!

What does matter is that you get back up on your horse and start looking for another filly to saddle up. Now, let's take the rejection factor out of the equation and fast forward past boy meets girl, first impressions, first phone conversation, etc. Let's jump to that inevitable, yet often awkward, event all relationships must endure . . . the first kiss.

"When it's right, you can't say who is kissing whom."
—Gregory Orr

The Perfect First Kiss

First off, there probably is no such thing! Why? All together now . . . because all women are different! What I have done, though, is taken a multitude of "perfect first kiss" descriptions and cobbled them together to form a singular "perfect first kiss" formula. At the very least, you won't come off as an amateur:

Step 1—Slowly move your hands to rest on either side of her face.

Step 2—Look into her eyes and tell her what you like about her and what attracts you to her.

Step 3—Slowly move your face closer to hers. Gently use your lips to kiss each of her lips individually.

Step 4—Continue kissing her lips while adding the action of gliding your tongue over her lips as you kiss them and gently pulling or sucking on each as you pull away and go for the other.

Step 5—While engaged in step 4, use your fingers to massage her earlobes, her head, or the back of her neck.

The average person spends 20,160 minutes kissing in their lifetime.

That's about as far as you should take it. If she's ready to play a serious game of tonsil hockey with you, she'll let you know it by either opening her mouth wider or trying to push her tongue past your lips. If that's the case, I say game on, of course!

So there you have my formula for the perfect first kiss. Unfortunately I can't do all the work; deciding when and where is all on you! More kissing tips are in chapter 15.

CHAPTER 13

Damsel in Distress

All women have different triggers that turn them on to a particular man. Unfortunately, something that might intrigue one woman could turn another completely off. Some women love men in uniforms, others have absolutely no interest in them. Some women are turned on by motorcycles, others stigmatize men who ride them. In general, though, there are a number of skills and types of expertise and knowledge that when demonstrated at the right time, in the presence of the right woman, will get you laid—or at least halfway there! Take a look at the following chart for a better understanding of what I'm talking about.

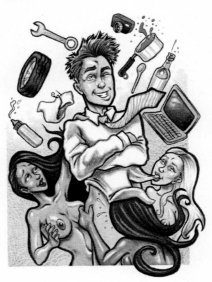

FEMALE TRIGGER	SKILL/EXPERTISE	COMMENT
Damsel in Distress	Tire Changing	If you're able to rescue a damsel in distress, she might look for ways to repay you for your heroics.
Damsel in Distress	Lock Picking	
Damsel in Distress	Hot-wire a Car	
Damsel in Distress	Computer Repair	There are some women who are very dependent upon their computers and will freak out if they're offline for any extended period of time. Having the skills to repair her computer could garner you hero status with her.
Maternal Instincts	Diaper Changing	Many women simply melt when they watch men handle babies with care and confidence. For those women, changing a dirty diaper without flinching makes you a superstar!
Intimacy	Photography	Some people say that cameras can look into the soul. The bond between photographer and client can be a very intimate one, without sex. That and the ability to make her look beautiful can be very rewarding.
Intimacy	Cooking	Being able to prepare her a good meal will give her the feeling that you have the ability to take care of her. Plus, some women are just wired like men in the sense that the way to their heart is through their stomach.
Intimacy	Dancing	Many women equate a man's ability to dance with his lovemaking skills. If you're not comfortable getting out on the dance floor, you need to teach yourself a signature dance move. Start watching some music videos and find a step you think you can handle. Practice it in the mirror until you're feeling comfortable enough to bust it out at the club.

continued

FEMALE TRIGGER	SKILL/EXPERTISE	COMMENT
Intimacy/Romance	Kissing	Considering that many women believe kissing to be more intimate than sucking a cock or tossing a salad, you can see how a man who's a great kisser can leave quite an impression.
Romance	Chivalry	Hey, for some women, chivalry is alive and well. Opening a door or pulling out a chair shows you're a considerate man, which might equate to a considerate lover in the minds of these women.
Romance	Play an Instrument (not the skin flute)	Why do you think musicians have all those hot groupies? Music has a seductive effect on women, and men who can make seductive music are at a definite advantage!
Romance	Ordering Wine/Food	Not only is this a take-charge type of action, but it also portrays a worldly, experienced man, which could equate to a worldly, experienced lover in the minds of some women.
Mystery	Magic	Some women love to be mystified. Also, many magic tricks give the magician reasons to touch and caress his female audience, which can add a level of intimacy.
Laughing	Joke Telling (see examples on the following pages)	Having the ability to make a woman laugh will usually result in her being more comfortable with you and relaxing her guard. The rest is up to you!

"Courtesy is as much a mark of a gentleman as courage."
—Teddy Roosevelt

It is said that playing the didgeridoo while pointing the instrument in close proximity to a woman's genital area can result in that woman actually achieving orgasms from the intense vibrations that emanate from the instrument.

Here are a few examples of some jokes I have found to be especially effective:

A Jewish mother unexpectedly finds her recently married daughter crying on her doorstep.

Jewish Mother: Honey, what's the matter?
Daughter: It's over, Mom, I left him!
Jewish Mother: But what about that beautiful house, those incredible vacations, and all that expensive jewelry?
Daughter: You don't understand, Mom. All he wants to do is have anal sex. When we got married my butthole was the size of a dime and now it's like a half dollar!
Jewish Mother: Sounds like you're making forty cents on the deal. I don't see the problem.

Again, for me the fact that this joke has an anal reference makes a woman's reaction to it of special interest to me. I'm more than comfortable using this type of language in front of strange women, whereas some of you may not be. If a woman wasn't comfortable with the language or subject matter, I would instantly know that I was sniffing around the wrong bush. You should select the jokes that you are most comfortable with!

Position your hand as if you were flipping her off with your pinkie and ring finger. Then, as you point to your fingers, ask her, "Do you know why it's impossible for you to masturbate with these two fingers?" When she asks why, you tell her, "Because they're mine!"

A woman went up to the bar in a quiet rural pub. She gestured alluringly to the bartender, who approached her immediately. She then seductively signaled that he should bring his face closer to hers. As he did, she gently caressed his full beard.

"Are you the manager?" she asked, softly stroking his face with both hands.

"Actually, no," he replied.

"Can you get him for me? I need to speak to him," she said, running her hands beyond his beard and into his hair.

"I'm afraid I can't," breathed the bartender. "Is there anything I can do?"

"Yes, I need you to give him a message," she continued, running her forefinger across the bartender's lip and slyly popping a couple of her fingers into his mouth and allowing him to suck them gently.

"What should I tell him?" the bartender managed to say.

"Tell him," she whispered, "there's no toilet paper, hand soap, or paper towels in the ladies' room."

Other Skills That Can Come in Handy

Bra Busting

I don't think I've unhooked a bra in at least five years. Mirna just doesn't wear them that often. When I was a younger man, though, I was a master of the one-handed titty release. I would actually practice the maneuver, between the ages of fourteen and sixteen, by strapping one of my mother's bras around the back of a chair. I became so good at unhooking those suckers, I could do it equally well with either hand. Give it a try, although

If you do like to cook you should know that chewing gum while peeling onions will keep you from crying.

I'm not recommending that you steal one of your mother's bras! You'll surprise yourself and your partner by how fast you're able to set those bound bosoms free!

Clubbing It

Getting turned away at the door of a nightclub when you're on a date can be extremely embarrassing and could get you shut out from another date. While I can't guarantee entry, I do have some suggestions to help avoid the potential humiliation.

You definitely want to dress to impress. It is safer to overdress than underdress in these situations. You want to avoid giving an asshole bouncer any visible reasons to deny you entry.

Before you approach, take a minute to observe the front door of the club. Try to identify the person in charge.

Now, grab your date by the hand and walk directly to the person in charge. Approach with a smile and casually ask how long the wait will be. If he quotes you anything longer than ten minutes, ask nicely where you should wait. If he tells you to stand in line, make sure to get in the right one. Most clubs have VIP and general-public lines, and you don't want to get stuck waiting in the VIP line only to be told to get in the back of the general-public line.

Find your place in line and get prepared to make your move. First take $20, $50, or $100 (the amount is up to you, but I will say that at a posh club in a major metropolitan city you'll be laughed at for a $20) and fold it up into the palm of your dominant hand. Excuse yourself from your date for a moment, put your hands in your pockets, and reapproach the same person you had previously talked to. This is what you say and do: First you say, "I know you said it would be ___ minutes, but it's my one-year anniversary and I really wanted to make my girl feel special tonight." Now, pulling the hand with the money out and extending it to him to shake hands, you say, "I would really appreciate it if there is anything you can do to help make that happen!" At this point, he will feel the money in his hand and hopefully adopt a new, much friendlier attitude. The next sound you hear should be that distinctive squish coming from between your date's legs as she becomes turned on by your ability to take charge

"Changing a diaper is a lot like getting a present from your grandmother—you're not sure what you've got but you're pretty sure you're not going to like it."—Jeff Foxworthy

and get things handled. Of course, the person could keep your money and still not let you in the club—but hey, without risk there's no reward!

Cleaning It

Imagine this scenario. You're with a date at a party at a friend's house. The two of you are mingling with the host and some other guests when someone bumps into your date, causing her to spill red wine on her blouse and the host's carpet. As one idiot runs for the club soda while your date is near tears, you step in to save the day. Ask the host for some hydrogen peroxide and some sort of fabric-appropriate soap, e.g. dishwashing liquid, liquid detergent, or rug shampoo. Mix three parts hydrogen peroxide with one part soap in a spray bottle or container of some kind. Using a towel wet with warm water, dab the spots and then spray or apply the mixture with a Q-tip—then watch the smiles appear as the stains disappear before everyone's eyes. This trick works on almost all stains, new or old, not just red wine. Just make sure the mixture you're using isn't more than a week old as it tends to lose potency over time.

CHAPTER 14

The Happy Pussy

What do women want in bed?

This is one of those questions that has perplexed man for centuries. What makes it so perplexing is that there are as many answers to it as there are women.

I always adopt the role of explorer during the first few sexual encounters with my new partner. I do this because I realize there is nothing more valuable to me at the start of a relationship than information. Some might call it ego, but I prefer to think of it as pride; I have always had the desire to please women, or to be more accurate, I want to be the best lover my partner has ever had. To achieve this, I know I have to learn as much about her as I possibly can. I approach those first few encounters like a student, if you will, always ready with a virtual pen and pad in my head to take extensive mental notes. I want to know about her turn-ons, turnoffs, thresholds, and fantasies. These first few encounters should be used to open lines of intimate communication and to test the waters through subtle exploration. Intimate communication is a key component of the emotional connection most women crave and can be established simply by letting her know how much you're enjoying your intimate time together.

I use my hands and mouth to test the waters, and my eyes and ears to gauge the results of those tests, so to speak. For every move I make, I'm taking mental notes of her reactions. A low moan, the slightest arching of her back or thrusting of her hips, the squeeze of her hand, her pussy getting wetter, etc. All these are indicators to me, generally indicators that I'm doing something right. It's just as important, however, to be aware of the negative indicators as well. For example, I'm fucking a woman and I feel her hands slightly pushing back against my hips. This tells me I'm probably going too deep and need to shorten my strokes for her in this particular position. You see, you just can't assume that because your last partner loved it balls-deep doggie style that your new partner will as well. It would be so much easier if each woman came with her own individual instruction manual, but they don't. That's why being a great lover isn't easy. You have to want to rock her world and you have to be willing to do what it takes to accomplish that!

My thirty-plus years of sexual experience have led me to develop a sexual philosophy of sorts.

I go into almost every sexual encounter, except, of course, for the quickie, with the idea that I am creating a private pleasure "oasis," because it is an acronym for the things I have found women want most in bed: orgasms, adventure, skills, intimacy, and sensitivity! These five things are so important, I beg you to repeat them one more time before we move on to examine each more closely:

Orgasms—This one seems a little obvious to me, but I'll say it anyway: All women want orgasms! However, if you haven't figured that one out by now, I don't know if this book can help you.

Adventure—I'm not suggesting that you have sex while skydiving at ten thousand feet, but I am suggesting you be aware of falling into a sexual routine, especially in longer relationships. I point this out because it is man's nature to stick with the tried-and-true and there are few worse places for sexual relationships to arrive at than Boresville, which sits right at the base of Mount Monotony! The point is, you can't go wrong if you assume at least 50 percent of the responsibility of keeping things fresh and exciting. I have more detailed suggestions on this in chapter 24, "Throw Her a Curveball."

Skills—This is the area where the men get separated from the boys. Because if you ain't got the skills, you won't rock her world. That being said, concentrating on skills alone, while ignoring the other areas, is a certain recipe for failure. Great lovers are versatile, intuitive, and well-rounded.

Being a great fuck is not the same as being a great lover. Even a guy without skills can occasionally get lucky and pair off with somebody inexperienced or inebriated enough to consider him a great fuck. There is no luck involved with being a great lover, as it is simply a matter of desire, knowledge, and effort. Well, maybe it's not so simple, but that's what it takes!

Intimacy—This one's probably the most difficult concept for men to get a grip on, myself included. It took me years to begin to understand all that was involved with this foreign concept. And I'm positive some of my past girlfriends would attest to this. I am confident, though, that I have learned a few things over the years that could be of value to you.

Intimacy is about communication. It is so important to establish a bedroom atmosphere in which both partners feel that they can say anything to each other in regard to sex and not be judged or laughed at or made to feel inadequate. This is not easy and requires being open and honest, and a touch of romance as well. While I do encourage open and honest communication at all times, I don't believe the bedroom is the best

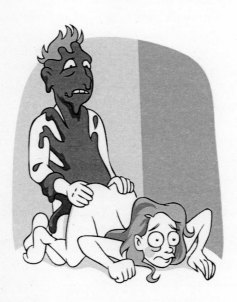

place for critiques of sexual performance. If she's doing something you don't like, subtly change things up and make a mental note to bring it up at another time, preferably a time when you are at ease and getting along well. When you do bring it up, make sure you are ready to mention something she does that you really like. Please notice, I said if she's doing something you don't *like*, "like" being the operative word. *Pain* is a whole 'nother story! If you're receiving a blow job and her teeth are making your cock feel like a discarded sausage being pecked by ravenous crows, for god's sake, man, say something!

Other than that, keep your mouth shut until later. She wants to hear you like the way her skin feels, how she turns you on, how you love her silver-dollar areolas or the birthmark on her sphincter. She wants to know how good she makes you feel when she's sucking your cock and she wants to hear your pleasure when you come inside her. Most of all, she wants to know she's special—to you!

Fore- and after-play are big parts of intimacy as well. Foreplay is all about kissing, touching, caressing, and licking. Many women will tell you they consider kissing a more intimate act than giving head or fucking. From the man's perspective, foreplay is his opportunity to set the tone of each encounter, his chance to let his partner know he means business. As a general rule, when it comes to foreplay, more is better! After-play is another tough one for men. It's not that we actually dislike it, it's just that our bodies aren't really cut out for it. We are basically preprogrammed to roll over and fall asleep after sex. Women, of course, are the exact opposite. They experience a euphoric revitalization of sorts and want to kiss, cuddle, and talk. Personally, I could fall asleep within thirty seconds of my last spurt of ejaculate. My way of compromising is to make sure I stay inside my partner, while continuing the kissing and caressing, until my cock gets completely soft and falls out of its resting place. This will usually buy me a few minutes of after-play credits before I head off to dreamland.

Sensitivity—I'm not just talking about being sensitive to her wants and needs, which is obviously very important. That is a matter of desire and effort, two things she will notice and appreciate immensely. You have to remember, men are the penetrators, women the penetrated. There is no place a woman feels more vulnerable or exposed than in the bedroom.

"Women are like phones. They like to be held, talked to, and touched, but push the wrong button and your ass is disconnected!"—Unknown

The place that offers the potential for pleasure and fantasy fulfillment offers the same potential for embarrassment, regret, and shame. Most of the potentially embarrassing situations that can and do happen during sex happen to women. It's how we react as men to each situation that dictates whether embarrassment, regret, or shame become part of the experience.

Think about it as I cite some examples:

Women can bleed or urinate uncontrollably during intercourse. Do you cry about your sheets and make an issue of it or do you man up, find a dry spot, and finish her off right?

Due to the pumping action of intercourse, air can get trapped in a woman's body and "farted" or "queefed" out, at exactly the wrong moment . . . that is, if you make it a wrong moment.

It is not uncommon for women to gag or even throw up while giving a man a blow job. Do you become noticeably grossed out or do you commend her on the attempted deep throat and offer to lend a hand to clean it up?

Do I even need to go into the potential for embarrassment with anal sex? Probably not, but I'm gonna do it anyway . . .

Once upon a time, when I was a young man of twenty-one, I was introduced to a girl named Alice by a close friend. There was instant chemistry between us. She was a slim five-foot-five blonde, with fair skin, big natural breasts, puffy nipples, beautiful blue eyes, and a great smile. When our mutual friend pointed out our mutual love of anal sex, the deal was sealed! The first time we had sex, she invited me to her parents' for a dinner party, took me upstairs, pulled out two Ecstasy tabs, and asked me to "fuck her butt" while her parents and their guests partied away downstairs. Obviously, I was more than thrilled to oblige.

The next time we got together, we went to a movie. We made out through the entire second half of the movie and I even finger-banged her to orgasm during the closing credits. As we pulled out of the theater parking lot in my '72 green Cadillac Coupe de Ville, Alice asked me to find a bathroom for her. Two blocks down, I pulled into a Taco Bell and watched Alice walk inside to get the key and disappear into the bathroom. We were on our way to a party at her friend's house, so I figured she was freshening up a bit. About five minutes after entering the bathroom, she poked her head out the door and motioned for me to come in. When I walked in, I was quite surprised to find Alice naked from the waist down, except for her heels, and bent over the sink waiting for me. I kissed her and then moved behind her, dropped to my knees, and ate her pussy. Soon I was pumping my cock into Alice from behind as we both watched ourselves in the cracked, graffiti-covered mirror.

As we were going at it, I noticed a small jar of Vaseline sitting on the sink. I asked if that was for what I thought it was for and she replied with a definite "You know it, baby! I want you to stick it in my butt!" She didn't have to ask twice. I pulled out of her pussy, lubed her ass up, and slowly entered Alice's anus. There might have been a few knocks at the door while we were going at it, but we couldn't have cared less. I had my hand between her legs playing with her clit and was whispering dirty things in her ear when she said, "Oh fuck, don't stop! I'm gonna come!" I didn't stop and she did come!

As I backed my head away from her ear and prepared for my own orgasm, I felt something dripping down my thighs. At the same time, Alice looked back at me and asked me to stop for a second. I pulled out and looked down at my thighs and at the back of her legs. It looked like we had just taken a stroll through waist-deep mud! I wanted to yell "Oh shit!" but resisted. Instead we looked at each other and laughed, and then she said it—"Oh shit!" She tried covering her ass with her hands as she was suddenly overcome by more of the "Hershey squirts." She took three steps in an attempt to get to the toilet before getting her heel caught in a floor drain and falling flat on her face.

I thought she might be hurt but she started laughing—the more she laughed, the more she farted and Hershey squirted all over the place. She was laughing so hard she had to crawl the rest of the way to the toilet. I started crying from laughing. If I hadn't been with Alice for the last two hours and known she only had popcorn and a Sprite, I might have suspected she had just participated in a burrito-eating contest!

At this point, I could have acted grossed out or disgusted, but the last thing I wanted to do was add to Alice's embarrassment in any way. Let's face it, she might have been laughing on the outside, but you knew she had to be crying on the inside. So instead of potentially killing the relationship by saying or doing something stupid, I volunteered to clean her up. It took every scrap of toilet paper and the toilet seat covers to get the job done, leaving nothing but water for me—and as for even attempting to clean up the bathroom, there was just no way. I just wanted to get the fuck out of there without getting arrested! Of course, it was my luck that ten thirty P.M. happened to be rush hour at the Taco Bell bathrooms. There were at least six people in line waiting and they didn't look happy. I can only imagine what they thought when they saw the bathroom. We speed-walked to the car and burned rubber out of the parking lot. It didn't take long, being in the confined space of my car, to realize that I might not have done as good a job as I thought I did cleaning us off. We decided to skip the party and head straight to Alice's house, where she looked in my eyes, thanked me, kissed me, and told me to call her in the morning—she said she owed me one.

I'm not sure if she was referring to the incident, the fact that I didn't get to come, or both. It didn't matter because I was on the receiving end of many more than "one" from Alice over the next couple of months—great experiences with a great girl that I might never have had the pleasure of if I had reacted differently that night in the Taco Bell bathroom.

Can you see how we as men are really in control of how each and every one of those potential embarrassments plays out via our reactions to them? These are the times when understanding and sensitivity are called

"It is not sex that gives the pleasure, but the lover."—Marge Piercy

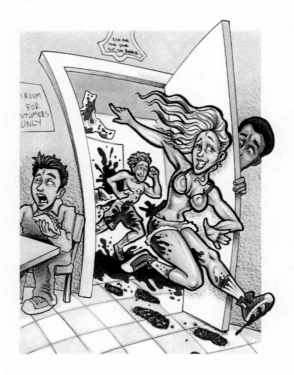

for and a sense of humor can't hurt. These are also the times that will let her know whether she's fucking a man or a mouse!

Ten Traits of Great Lovers

Many men assume that being a great lover is about the number of "parlor tricks" they know or the size of their cock, but that is far from the truth. Moves might earn you the title of great lay, which is not necessarily the same as being considered a great lover.

Ask a hundred women to define a great lover and you'll probably get at least eighty different answers. However, if you were to examine the definitions given by those one hundred women you would find some distinct commonalities. In fact, if you listen closely, you will find that being a great lover boils down to three big-picture factors.

"Bed is the poor man's opera."—Italian proverb

- Attitude
- Behavior
- Knowledge

Over the course of the last three decades, I have had thousands of intimate discussions with women. Based on those conversations, I have expanded the list of common factors above into a more detailed profile I call "Ten Traits of Great Lovers":

1. **A Curious and Open Attitude Toward Sex**
   Curiosity leads to learning, which leads to knowledge, which is the ultimate sexual power! Having an open attitude toward new sexual experiences will not only give you the opportunity to learn more about your sexual self but also helps strengthen the bond between you and your partner via the inevitable sharing of first-time experiences together. It also means that you don't judge others when it comes to their individual turn-ons and turnoffs.

2. **Desire to Give Pleasure**
   If you don't consider yourself a top-notch lover, which I have to assume is the case considering you're reading this book, you probably fit into one of the following three categories:

   - Lazy
   - Selfish
   - Don't know any better

Now, in my opinion, the first two are inexcusable and the third is the reason I wrote this thing! The good news is that if you do fit into one of the first two categories, you obviously recognize it or you wouldn't be reading this now. The simple truth is you have to want to be a great lover before you can actually be one. As you will learn, so much about being a great lover is about desire and effort: the desire to rock her world and the willingness to put in the effort that it takes. A woman wants to know that you want to please her and are ready to do whatever it takes to accomplish it!

3. Knowledge of Your Anatomy

The more you know about your body and how it works, the better! This self-knowledge is beneficial in a variety of ways. Knowing the time of day your erections are strongest, knowing what type of stimulation works best to get you hard, knowing what your stimulation thresholds are (how long you can keep fucking after you receive that first orgasmic signal before you reach the point of no return), and knowing your needed recovery time between erections, among other things, are all invaluable bits of knowledge that will inevitably be of use to a sexually active man—especially to a man who yearns to be a great lover.

4. Knowledge of the Female Anatomy

Nothing impresses a woman more than a man who knows how the female body works as well or better than she does, even if some won't admit it and a smaller percentage might say they find it intimidating. Believe me, once you demonstrate the benefits of your knowledge to her, the timid will become bold and brave. It's important to note that great lovers realize that a general expertise in the female anatomy is not enough. That's because they never forget that all women are different. They take on the additional responsibility of learning as much as possible about their partner's specific body and how it responds to sexual stimuli.

5. Being a Good Listener

One way or another, a woman will tell you what she likes and dislikes.

"All men are the same. They're only interested in fucking you and they don't care whether you're happy or sad. They just want to get on with their business in and out of bed, and they make you feel that you don't count except as their sex toy."
—Cameron Diaz

The problem is they don't always use their mouths to actually say the words. That's why you have to know that it takes more than good hearing to be a good listener. Women speak with their bodies as well. A hand against your hips as you're pounding away from above is probably her way of saying you're penetrating too deeply. On the other hand, if she takes her ankles and starts wearing them as earrings, it's probably her way of telling you she's ready for everything you've got to give her. This may have as much to do with conditioning as anything. We men don't necessarily make it easy for women to verbally communicate the types of intimate information they want us to know and that we need to know. We either haven't shown a willingness to have the conversations or we don't respond to those conversations in the bedroom. One obvious reason both men and women have difficulty with intimate sexual conversations is because a majority of us have been discouraged from having them since early childhood: "We don't talk about those things" or "You don't need to know that" being the most common responses to most of our sexual inquiries. Obviously, there are many things that she can't communicate with body alone and she will inevitably open up to you over time. It will be up to you to show her that you're receptive and, most importantly, that you're listening. Ultimately, the only way to prove you're listening is through your actions. A great lover realizes that intimate conversations are the key to gaining the type of carnal knowledge that will be invaluable during sex and, knowing this, makes every effort to initiate these conversations, which in turn give him the opportunity to show her what a good listener he is. Don't underestimate the number of women who will directly relate how much a man cares for her to how well that man listens to her.

6. Displays Sensitivity

Great lovers will put their partner's needs ahead of their own. They don't pressure their partners into doing things they're not comfortable with and don't make them feel guilty for not wanting to do something. Great lovers turn those seemingly unavoidable embarrassments—a fart, a queef, bleeding, urinating, etc.—into humor, or at the very least handle them in a mature manner.

7. Genuinely Likes Women

There are many men out there who just don't like women, period! While I'm sure some have compelling reasons, I guarantee that a man who doesn't truly love women is not going to be considered a great lover by any woman. Women can sense the hate. That's not to say women-haters won't get laid. They will, but they'll either be paying for it or fucking a woman who has an equal hatred for men. That's called a grudge fuck, and while it's quite common, this is probably the last time I'll be mentioning those two words, as they have no place in a book like this. Great lovers appreciate all of their partner, not just their orifices.

8. Good Grooming and Hygiene

I have never met a woman who said she didn't appreciate a man who grooms his garden. It doesn't stop at your cock, balls, or ass, however. Women take notice of ear and nose hair, finger- and toenails, teeth, breath, hairstyle, manner of dress, facial hair, armpits, etc. While it may seem like a lot to worry about, paying attention to these things shows a woman you value yourself and therefore you are worthy of her time. It also allows the woman to relax and be adventurous knowing, for example, that your fingernails are clean and smooth when you insert them inside her and she won't be attacked by any dingleberry monsters if she wants to explore your ass. An added benefit is that your partner will be forced to be especially conscious of her own personal grooming and hygiene needs, as few women will accept the thought of being less well groomed than their man.

9. Strong Hands and Finger Dexterity

Fingers and hands are as important to a skilled lover as they are to a concert pianist. Strong hands and dexterous fingers used in concert with the knowledge you'll have when you've finished this book will put you on the fast track. Think about how often they come into play during a typical sexual encounter:

- They're used every time you touch, massage, grab, and squeeze her
- They're used specifically to stimulate breasts and nipples
- They're used specifically to stimulate the clitoris

> "The first duty of love is to listen."—Paul Tillich

- They're used specifically to stimulate the G-spot and vagina
- They're used specifically to stimulate the anus
- They're used to support yourself when on top of her

STRENGTH

- Squeezing—Using a tennis or handball, squeeze it and release until your hand starts to ache. Make sure you exercise each hand equally. It's easy to do just about any time and you can never do it too much. Of course, there are products specifically made to help strengthen your hands that can be purchased at any sporting goods outlet.
- Hanging—Grab a chin-up bar, lift your legs off the floor, and hold on for dear life as long as you can. Try to hold on for a little longer each time.
- Pinching—Take a weight plate in each hand and hold them at your sides for as long as you can by pinching them between your thumb and four fingers. Progress can be achieved by increasing the weight and hold times. You should start with a weight you can hold no longer than twenty to thirty seconds.

DEXTERITY

- Paper Shuffle—Place a sheet of paper in one hand and crumple it up into a small ball using that one hand only. Then uncrumple the paper and repeat with the other hand.
- Finger Lift—Place your palm and fingers on a flat surface and practice lifting each finger individually while the others remain flat and still. Once you have perfected this, you can work to improve your speed and vary the pattern of your finger lifting.
- Pen Spinning—This is not only a great way to improve your finger dexterity but could be your only shot at becoming a professional athlete by participating in next year's Pen Spinning

World Cup. Pen spinning involves spinning and/or twirling a pen or pencil between and around your fingers and hands. I highly recommend you try learning tricks like the "pen roll," the "thumb around," the "sonic reverse," and the "double charge combo." If you are interested, check out pentrix.com for all the information you need to get started.

10. Endurance

I'm talking about both cardiovascular and muscular endurance. As you can imagine, most of your major muscle groups are engaged in one way or another during a typical sex session. Some of these muscle groups are used more than others and there are specific exercises you can do to improve your sexual fitness.

Aside from your hands, these are the parts of the body that take on the greatest workload during sex.

Lower back	Stomach	Heart
Hips	Shoulders	Chest
Thighs	Arms	Wrists

Considering that and drawing upon my experience as a personal trainer, I have devised a workout regimen I call the "circuit for sexual fitness" that I recommend be done three times weekly. It is designed for you to be able to do it practically anywhere.

You will be exercising your heart because you will do each exercise immediately after the other, not resting until after you've completed the entire circuit of seven exercises. You should repeat the circuit three to five times, with a two to three minute rest between circuits. Here are a few other things you should know:

- When you perform an exercise to failure, you're either completing repetitions of a movement until you simply can't do any more, or you're holding a particular position until you can't hold it any longer.
- Breathing correctly is very important while exercising. You

EXERCISE	BODY PARTS INVOLVED

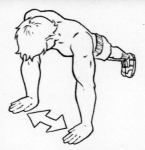

One set of push-ups to failure — Shoulder, upper arms, wrists, hands, chest

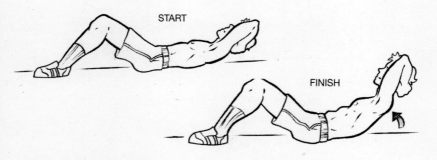

START

FINISH

One set of crunches to failure — Stomach, lower back

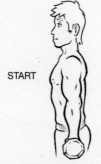 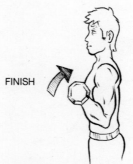

START

FINISH

One set of bicep curls to failure — Hands, wrists, forearms, upper arms

EXERCISE   **BODY PARTS INVOLVED**

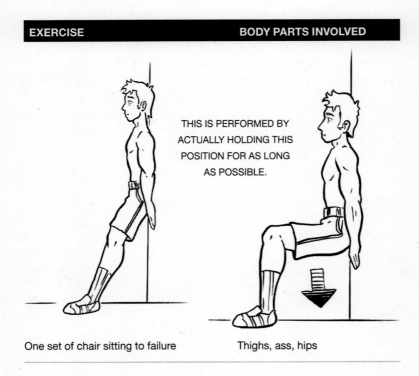

THIS IS PERFORMED BY ACTUALLY HOLDING THIS POSITION FOR AS LONG AS POSSIBLE.

One set of chair sitting to failure   Thighs, ass, hips

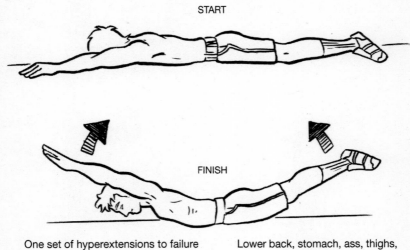

START

FINISH

One set of hyperextensions to failure   Lower back, stomach, ass, thighs, hips

EXERCISE	BODY PARTS INVOLVED

START   FINISH

One set of wrist curls to failure   Wrists, forearms, hands

START

FINISH

One set of pelvic thrusts to failure   Lower back, stomach, ass, thighs, hips

should always be exhaling when exerting and inhaling when returning to your starting position.

Warning

Some of you will need the following words of caution. Just because you are called a great lover, or a great fuck, for that matter, doesn't mean you have what it takes to be a porn star. Trust me when I say I've wasted more time in my life waiting for so-called male performers to get an erection or blow their load than I have in California traffic. If it really was as easy as it looks, don't you think many more guys would be doing it? After all, it would seem like a dream job to many—getting paid to get laid! Yet, if you watch adult movies with any frequency, you'll notice the same twenty to thirty guys recycled in almost every movie. That's because being a male performer is the most difficult job in the adult film industry.

Fucking on camera is not like fucking in the comfortable confines of your own bedroom. Something just happens to a majority of guys when they hear the word "action." Sometimes if I listen closely, I can hear the whoosh of blood rushing away from the male performer's genitals. There are few sights more pathetic than a man struggling to get an erection in a room full of cast and crew. The most consistent and successful male performers share a unique set of traits—an abundant supply of natural testosterone flowing through their body, the ability to relax when having sex with strangers in front of a crowd of more strangers, and the ability to summon visually stimulating images to their mind's eye at will.

Again, I don't care what women have told you—you're so hot, your dick is huge, you rocked her world—the odds are you don't have what it takes to be a porn star. Age, race, height, weight—none of it matters when compared to your ability to achieve and maintain an erection under duress. Think

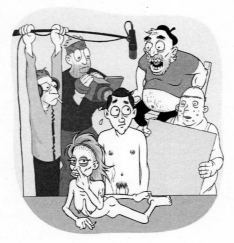

"Alright, then . . . *get a boner!!*"

"I've often said, the only thing standing between me and greatness is me."—Woody Allen

about it for a moment—you're being told when, how, where, with whom, and how long to have sex with people you may or may not be physically attracted to. And if you don't like something about your working conditions, nobody gives a shit! If you had a pussy and a great set of tits they might, but you don't! Male performers are essentially props that need to be able to get it up, get it in, and get it off on command—period. The fact is, 95 percent of all new male performers can't hack it. Just take a look at Ron "Hedgehog" Jeremy, one of the most successful of all time, and you'll understand what I am saying about looks and body shape being unimportant!

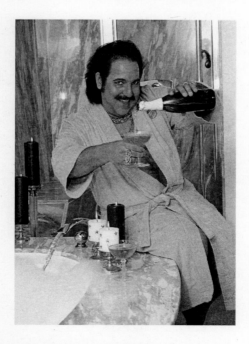

Despite his rubenesque figure, abundance of body hair, and malodorous underarms, Ron is continually cast with and, I might add, many times requested by the most beautiful girls in the adult industry despite the fact that there are a plethora of younger, much more aesthetically pleasing male "specimens" available for hire. The reason is simple: Porn is a business. In business, time equals money. And nothing, I mean nothing short of a police raid can cause an adult-movie producer or porn starlet to waste more time than a "dud" masquerading as a "stud."

CHAPTER 15

Straight from the Kitty's Mouth

You have no idea how much time I've spent thinking about what I should or should not include in this book. I continuously went over the table of contents debating what should stay and what should go or what was missing. I want to cover every angle of every topic but I know that's not possible and would bore the shit out of you. Yet I have nightmares of reviewing the book after it's been printed and finding I've left out something important. Then one very late night while staring at the table of contents, it hit me! I was missing a very important angle—the female perspective. You know the old saying about getting it straight from the horse's mouth: I thought the best way to go about it was to just throw it out there to the general female public. I used my Internet resources to blast the following questionnaire to all interested females:

How do you like to be kissed?
How do you like your pussy eaten?
How do you like to be fucked?

I received hundreds of answers and quoted the most interesting for you in the following pages. I hope you'll find the answers as interesting as I did.

Kissing

"I like to be kissed slow, not too soft but don't swallow my face either. Start by kissing my lips softly, adding pressure as you go along. Nibble and bite on the lips a little and then add some tongue."

"I like for a man to kiss me passionately with his tongue circling mine slow and easy . . . occasionally capturing my tongue and sucking on it slowly and then biting my bottom lip gently and delicately."

"I like when a man will come right up to my face, look at me, lightly lick my lips, and then pull away. Then right after he will do it again and then slip his tongue in my mouth."

"Very soft and sensual with just a little touch of the man's tongue to begin with as a little tease."

"The hottest, most erotic kind of kiss starts off light with some barely-there tongue, then gets gradually deeper, until there is no air between our mouths anymore and our tongues can play with each other without any predictable pattern."

"My favorite way to be kissed is when my man grabs my face with his hands and kisses me nice and slow with his tongue."

"At first kiss me gently, taste my lips and nibble softly. Then devour me, kiss me with passion!"

"What really turns me on is when he pulls away from me, holds my head in both his hands, and looks at me in the middle of a passionate kiss . . . then comes back in for more."

Pussy Eating

"I want him to tease my clit through my panties with his fingers. I want him to pull my panties aside and start teasing my lips by brushing his lips softly against them. Then he slides my lips open with his tongue using a soft fluttering, licking motion which leads to a wet, full, wide tongue licking me up and down, side to side, and around my clit in circles. Finish me off by softly but firmly sucking on my clit while his fingers stroke inside me and I'm in heaven."

"I cannot explain to men enough, it is not dog water in a dog bowl! Don't just lick it and look at me for approval! For god's sake, love the pussy with all you've got. The tongue is a strong muscle, use it!"

"I love when a man sticks his tongue deep in my pussy like he was licking the inside of an ice cream cone."

"Licking and sucking is always good but variation is key! Don't forget to use your hands as we have two openings that need to be filled while you're doing the dirty!"

"I like it licked and sucked on a lot. Put your whole mouth over it and kiss it for heaven's sake!"

"I love it when a guy teases me first and really gets me going before he dives in."

"Recently a guy actually covered my whole pussy with his mouth right as I was getting ready to get off and started humming while flicking my clit with his tongue. Damn, sent me so far over, was the best move I've ever had!"

"I like for a man to run his fingers inside my wet pussy lips, spreading them gently. Then he takes my clit into his mouth and slowly sucks on it while he inserts one, then two fingers inside me—slowly finger-fucking me while he is licking and sucking my clit. I also love it when a man sucks my clit between his lips and hums!"

"But the thing I like the most is the side-to-side motion. It's a little more difficult than the standard flickering-of-the-tongue technique but it really takes me there!"

"It is best when a man starts at my knees and works his way up slooooooowly, kissing and licking me all the way to my pussy. This will drive me nuts. See, sometimes the wanting is the best part! It makes you wanna take his head and jam it in!"

"Nothing feels better than being eaten out, sucking cock, and having your asshole fingered!"

"I love it when my partner opens my legs and licks around my pussy

first, teasing me. I love to be licked from my taint to the top of
my clit."

"I like the slow long licks and suckles and, of course, sticking your
tongue in as far as possible. Eat my pussy and make me cum
until your lips and chin are covered with my juice and then
kiss me . . . fuck that's hot!!"

Fucking

"The dirty girl who lives inside my body really loves it hard, fast,
and please, please bite my neck, back, and ass!"

"Pumping too fast is horrible . . . a nice rhythm is so great! Not too
fast and not too slow, but most men don't realize that during
sex there are other areas to stimulate, i.e., nipples, ass, clit, etc."

"When I'm just getting to know someone, I want him to be curious
about my body and interested in finding out what feels good to
me. He should take his time. I want to have the time to find
out what he likes as well."

"Once I'm wet, I love for a man to tease my pussy just a bit with the
head of his cock, just going a little deeper each time, and then
surprising me with one really deep thrust!"

"I like my ass all the way in the air with the side of my face resting
on the bed. This is my favorite because I like the feeling of
balls hitting my pussy as a cock thrusts in and out."

"As you're getting ready to cum, pull my hair and kiss me deep and
hard as you pump it into me!"

"I love for a man to start out slow and deep when fucking me,
rubbing his hands up and down my body, occasionally
caressing my face and kissing me deeply as he picks up the
pace."

"I like my hair pulled, my ass slapped, and nipple play during
fucking."

"I like it when he bites my lips, holds my face, and kisses me hard,
while thrusting it all the way in."

"Guys, don't just keep one rhythm or pace—work that pussy! Leave

a gaping hole as wide as the width of your cock! Own that
pussy!"
"I really like being grabbed and touched a lot while I'm being
fucked."

Overall, I found that the women seemed to be in general agreement
on quite a few common themes. The following stood out the most to me:

- Almost every woman who answered stated a preference for
starting slow and building up the pace and action, whether
they were talking about kissing, oral sex, or fucking.
- Foreplay is a must for 91 percent of the women who answered.
- 87 percent of the responses included mention of the word
"tease" or "teasing" in a positive way.
- 68 percent of the women mentioned how they like a man to
hold their head or touch their face while kissing.
- 61 percent of the responses mentioned the desire for eye contact during sex.
- 44 percent of the women said they enjoyed when a man inserted his fingers in her pussy during oral sex.
- 83 percent of the women said they liked their body touched a
lot during sex.
- 90 percent of the women who responded stated they prefer to be
placed in a variety of positions during a single sexual encounter.
- 49 percent of the women stated they wanted to know that the
guy was enjoying himself.

Surprisingly, only *one* woman mentioned anything in regard to the
size of the cock she preferred, stating that anything less than six inches is
a waste of time for her. Trust me, she'll change her tune as soon as she
meets a guy with a five-inch cock who's read this book!

In that same questionnaire, I asked women to tell me about things men
do that they don't like. From those responses, I picked out the twenty-
eight most common complaints and have listed them for you below:

1. Premature ejaculation
2. Sloppy kissing
3. No romance
4. Routine sex
5. Entering her before she's ready (not enough foreplay)
6. Rough touch
7. Too hairy
8. Not washing before sex (smelly balls or ass)
9. Going straight for the clit during oral sex
10. Undressing her clumsily
11. Spanking her without permission
12. Talking about the prowess of ex-lovers
13. Not being able to find the G-spot
14. Forcing her head down on your cock
15. Coming in her mouth without warning
16. Leaving hickeys
17. Asking her if she had an orgasm
18. Apologizing for the size of your penis
19. Crushing her during sex
20. Not cleaning up after sex
21. Dropping a *used* condom on the floor
22. Rolling eyes or sighing when eating pussy
23. Licking pussy in the same spot for extended periods of time (unless you're seeing a positive reaction)
24. Licking pussy like a lollipop
25. Being silent during sex
26. Jackhammer fucking
27. Chapped lips
28. Bad breath

It's probably not a coincidence that every one of those complaints is addressed in this book in one way or another. I do believe this list can serve as a great guide to what not to do until you have become more familiar with any particular partner. For example, it is very possible that you might meet a woman who gets off on having her head handled like a steering wheel while a hard cock is driven down her throat; however, it's

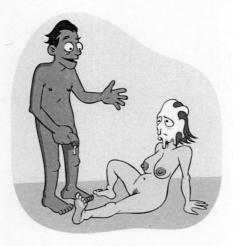

"Well, of course I didn't *warn* you.
If I'd warned you, you would have *ducked!*"

probably best to err on the side of caution and wait until she asks for that. Once she knows you are willing to do whatever it takes to rock her world, trust me, she'll eventually let you know what she likes, whatever that may be. (Hopefully anal!)

CHAPTER 16

Here She Comes!

There are six types of orgasms that a woman can enjoy. Each is unique and dependent on the type of stimuli used. Sadly, most women won't have the chance to sample all six during the course of their lifetime for a variety of reasons, including mental or physical obstacles and inept male partners. As a matter of fact, most women don't even know there are six different orgasms possible for them to experience! Imagine if you were the man who was able to introduce women to new types of orgasms. Imagine what a powerful impression that could make on a woman. Now, stop imagining, because you are about to become that guy. Before we get to the different types of orgasms, I think it's important to understand the female sexual response cycle, or, in simpler terms, what happens to a woman during orgasm. Sex therapists Masters and Johnson identified four distinct phases that are part of a continuous cyclical pattern within the sexual response cycle.

1. Excitement Phase
   - Begins with physical and/or mental stimulation
   - Blood rushes to her sexual anatomy, causing lubricated vagina, swollen clitoris, enlarged labia, elevated uterus, and swollen breasts
   - Heart rate and blood pressure increase
   - Muscles get tense
2. Plateau Phase
   - Occurs as stimulation increases

- Upper two-thirds of vagina expand
- Uterus further elevates to allow easier passage of sperm into fallopian tubes

3. Orgasmic Phase
   - She experiences powerful contractions of the vaginal, uterine, anal, and lower abdominal muscles
   - Blood pressure, heart rate, and respiratory rates reach peak
4. Resolution Phase
   - Blood in genitals begins to drain
   - Blood pressure, heart rate, and respiratory rates decrease
   - Uterus returns to normal position
   - Breasts decrease in size

Okay, now that you have an idea of what she's experiencing during orgasm, let's talk about the different types she can experience.

Six Types of Orgasms

1. Vulva Orgasm—This is triggered by clitoral stimulation.
2. Uterine Orgasm—This is triggered by vaginal intercourse.
3. Vulva/Uterine Orgasm—This is triggered by a combination of clitoral stimulation and simultaneous vaginal intercourse.
4. Anal Vulval—This is triggered by a combination of clitoral stimulation and anal intercourse.
5. Vaginal G-spot—This is triggered by G-spot stimulation achieved through vaginal penetration. Female ejaculation can accompany this type of orgasm.
6. Anal G-spot—This is triggered by G-spot stimulation achieved through anal penetration. Again, female ejaculation can result from this type of penetration.

A pig's orgasm lasts for thirty minutes.

Three Ways to Classify Orgasms

Standard Orgasm—This is an orgasm in which climax is the result. The climax is extremely pleasurable for a woman but does not last long, and there is often a physical or mental letdown period immediately afterward. The climax is usually a series of vaginal contractions that can last anywhere from several seconds to half a minute.

Multiple Orgasm—This is a series of standard orgasms experienced by a woman over a short period of time. Think of it like an orgasmic rollercoaster ride, climbing the peak of ecstasy, down the other side, then rushing to the top of "Mount Climax" and back down again.

Extended Orgasm—This is a single orgasm that lasts for an extended period of time. With no peaks and valleys, the woman "sticks" in climax mode and maintains that level of pleasurable sensation for anywhere from ten minutes to over an hour in some cases.

Now, not only do you have the ability to educate her about the variety of orgasms she can potentially experience, but soon you will have the skills to introduce her to them all personally! Unless . . . your partner is not able to achieve orgasm. This can be very discouraging for both people involved as it can lead to feelings of sexual inadequacy and cause distress within the relationship. There are many possible reasons why a woman can't achieve orgasms. Let's discuss some of the more common ones.

Covered or Hooded Clitoris—Some women have excessive amounts of tissue that actually cover the clitoris to the point of severely limiting the amount of surface area that can be stimulated, which in turn directly af-

The term "clitoris" is derived from a Greek word meaning "little hill."

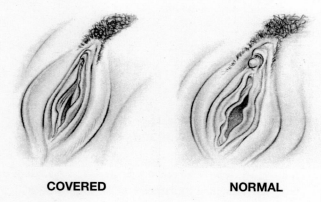

COVERED   **NORMAL**

fects that woman's ability to achieve orgasm. Take a look at these illustrations to see the difference between a covered clitoris and a normal clitoris.

The good news is that there is a relatively simple one-hour surgical procedure that can be performed to correct this called a clitoral unhooding or hoodectomy. If surgery is recommended make sure the surgeon is experienced in performing the procedure. It's a simple surgery but a very delicate area.

Medication—Certain medications but especially antidepressants can interfere with a woman's ability to achieve orgasm.

Female Sexual Arousal Disorder (FSAD)—FSAD is diagnosed by the following symptoms:

Inability to achieve orgasm
Inability to produce vaginal lubrication
Decreased libido or lack of sexual desire

There are both emotional and physical causes of FSAD:

Communication problems within relationship
Lack of affection within relationship
Lack of emotional intimacy within relationship

Depression
Diabetes or heart disease
Restrictive upbringing regarding sex
Fatigue or stress
Negative/traumatic sexual experience

Other FSAD-related illnesses include:

Sexual Aversion Disorder—Individuals actively avoid sexual genital contact. Women usually report feelings of fear, anxiety, or disgust when presented with opportunities for intimacy.
Hypoactive Sexual Desire Disorder—Individuals have decreased sexual fantasies and a lack of desire for sexual activity.
Orgasmic Cephalgia—Individuals experience severe headaches around the point of orgasm. The pain interferes with the woman's desire to continue engaging in the sexual activity.

Dealing with any of these issues that I have described can be very

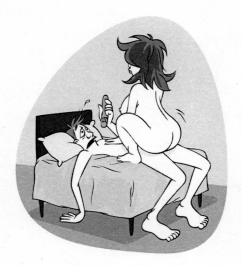

"I'll never make it—
you'll have to go on without me."

Forty-six percent of women who can't achieve orgasm blame the condition on their own negative self-image.

According to a survey of 15,000 women, only 9 percent said they are assured of reaching orgasm every time they have sex.

stressful and emotionally draining for both individuals involved in the relationship. Thankfully, with proper treatment, the majority of physical and emotional sexual dysfunctions can be overcome. They are matters for qualified professionals, though. Many times the best thing you could possibly do for a partner is recommend and encourage her to seek professional help! At the end of the day, it could turn out that you are the one man who was patient and supportive enough to help her get over this hump and discover her inner freak.

CHAPTER 17

Thar She Blows!

Even though it is almost twenty-five years ago now, I still remember the day quite vividly. My girlfriend Cristi and I were attending a swingers' convention in Las Vegas. It was day one, and we were relaxing by the pool when we were approached by one of the couples we had been talking with earlier— Vinny and Jackie from New Jersey. Jackie was twentysomething, cute, and brunette, with the muscular body of a gymnast. She was almost the exact opposite of Cristi, a five-foot-nine blonde with large breasts and a lean body. They proceeded to invite us up to their room to get better acquainted.

Cristi and I arrived at the room within twenty minutes. There we were greeted by Vinny and Jackie and introduced to another couple, Pam and Anthony. Pam was a very pretty blond exotic dancer from Detroit. Soon, the three girls were on the bed together, kissing and touching one another in various combinations while us guys took pictures or videotaped them. It quickly became apparent to me that Jackie and Pam had hooked up before, but they made sure that Cristi felt more than welcome!

As the action progressed, a large plug-in vibrator was introduced and Jackie quickly became the focus of attention. She lay flat on her back, with knees bent and spread open. She instructed Pam to start finger-fucking her and Cristi to sit on her face as she placed the head of the vibe on her clitoris. At the same time, Vinny grabbed me by the shoulder and pulled me closer to the action as he said, "You don't wanna miss dis!" My first thought was that this wiseguy thought I was some kind of amateur. I mean, did this dude think I had never seen women go at it before? However, it didn't take me long to figure out Vinny didn't mean what I thought he meant. Jackie's face started to contort and she told Pam, "Get ready, baby, I'm almost there!" Her words seemed to motivate Pam to move her fingers faster, which caused Jackie to yell out, "I'm gonna come!"

As soon as she heard that, as if it was a cue, Pam pulled her fingers out of Jackie and, well, I couldn't believe my eyes. Gush after gush of clear liquid exploded from Jackie's pussy. She literally hit the ceiling and everything and everyone that was near the bed. Neither Cristi nor I had any idea what we had just witnessed—other than that it was extremely hot!

As Jackie showed both girls her appreciation with her oral skills, I was left to contemplate this new discovery. Later, when I told the story to friends, I was met with calls of "Bullshit!" What I didn't know at the time was how much controversy there was surrounding the subject of female ejaculation and for how long the controversy has existed. Then, with my curiosity piqued, I began to seek out all the information I could about what I had witnessed.

The concept of female ejaculation and the existence of the G-spot have been debated since 1950, when Dr. Ernest Grafenberg published his paper "The Role of Urethra in Female Orgasm." He was the first person to

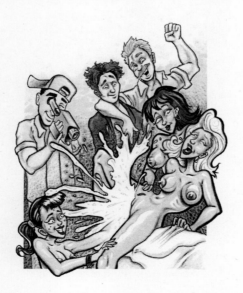

make mention of "an erotic zone that always could be demonstrated on the anterior wall of the vagina along the course of the urethra." This zone has since become known as the G-spot among believers. The "G," of course, is a tribute to Dr. Grafenberg. In that same paper, he also refers to female ejaculation: "If there is the opportunity to observe the orgasm of such women, one can see that large quantities of a clear, transparent fluid are expelled not from the vulva, but out of the urethra it gushes. At first I thought that the bladder sphincter had become defective by the intensity of the orgasm. Involuntary expulsion of urine is reported in sex literature. In the cases observed by us, the fluid was examined and it had no urinary character. I am inclined to believe that [urine] reported to be expelled during female orgasm is not urine, but only secretions of the intraurethral glands correlated with the erotogenic zone along the urethra in the anterior vaginal wall."

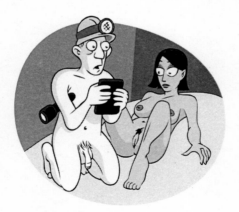

"No good—your G-spot
doesn't even show up on my GPS maps."

I know it's pretty detached and clinical, but I think it's interesting to read it as it was first presented to the scientific and medical communities back in 1950—almost sixty years ago. I would pay a lot to be able to travel back in time and observe Dr. Grafenberg at work. Forget Alfred Kinsey; I want to see this guy's life brought to the big screen!

Even though Dr. Grafenberg's findings have since been confirmed by other researchers, there are still professionals who will dispute the notion of female ejaculation and the existence of the G-spot. For example, I cannot sell my movies that contain depictions of female ejaculation in the U.K. or parts of Canada. This is because the censor boards that approve movies in these places claim there is not enough evidence to support the existence of female ejaculation and continue to label these scenes as depictions of urination! What can I say, the world is full of closed-minded morons and the rest of us suffer!

Take it from a man who's had numerous females ejaculate all over him and observed numerous others gush with glee: Female ejaculation does exist, and if you pay attention to what you read, you might get to experience it firsthand.

How to Find Her G-spot

What should you feel for? You are trying to find a quarter-sized oval area of slightly thicker/rougher-feeling tissue. The spot will swell and harden as your lady becomes more aroused. As Dr. Grafenberg described, the spot is felt through the anterior, or top, wall of the vagina. It is located directly behind the pubic bone and around the urethra, approximately one to three inches inside the vagina.

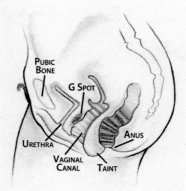

One thing to keep in mind: While the location of her G-spot never changes, you may have to change the way you locate it depending on the position her body is in. You should use one (index) or two (index and middle) fingers when attempting to locate and stimulate her G-spot. Here are three best positions to access her G-spot:

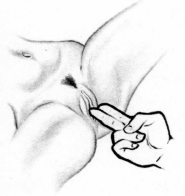

Missionary—When she is on her back, you would insert your finger(s) palm-up and apply upward pressure once you locate her spot. Also, there are times when you might find it helpful to use your free hand to place a downward pressure on her abdomen, just slightly above where her stomach meets her pubic bone. This will actually push her G-spot down to meet your probing fingers.

Doggie Style—When she is on her hands and knees, you would insert your finger(s) palm-down and apply downward pressure once you locate her spot.

Spoon—When she is on her side, you would insert your fingers sideways and apply lateral pressure to the anterior wall once you locate her spot.

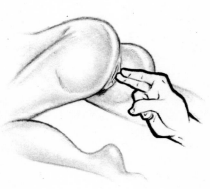

What to Do Once You Find It

I always prefer using two fingers, as I feel I get better leverage, and believe me when I say that with some women you need all the leverage you can get! Because as I've said before and will definitely say again, all women are different. This includes how much pressure they need applied to their G-spot and for that matter the actual size of their G-spot. Anyway, after you've inserted your fingers, there are three types of motions that seem to be particularly effective for stimulating her spot.

Come Hither

THE COME-HITHER

1.

2.

3. BACK TO #1 and repeat as necessary (til she comes—again and again—or until carpal tunnel sets in!)

THE FLUTTER

1.

2.

3. REPEAT back 'n' forth these bad boys til she can't take any more!

Flutter

THE SHUFFLE

1.

2.

3. VARIATION
Adding small circles can get Big results!

Shuffle

No matter what motion or combination of motions you're using, you will notice her spot enlarge and the pressure her pussy is putting on your fingers increase as she becomes more aroused. During the moment right before she is about to orgasm, you will start to feel as if her vagina is trying to expel or spit your fingers out—it is! Resist for a few seconds and then pull them out, as this will allow her to release any fluids without any impediment.

Play Options

1. You could always substitute a sex toy for your fingers, specifically one that is shaped for G-spot stimulation.
2. You could always incorporate simultaneous clitoral stimulation by adding a vibrator or a touch of oral sex to the action, just like Jackie did right before the tsunami gushed from her pussy.

What to Expect

Remember, every woman will respond differently to G-spot stimulation. Some can ejaculate within a few minutes from being finger-banged properly; others can take twenty minutes or more and need a vibrator with 300 horsepower to complement the G-spot stimulation. Some find it easier to ejaculate when on all fours, while others prefer to stand on their heads. Because of this, experimentation is key. Experimentation is the true method of gaining knowledge, and I've already spoken of how valuable and important knowledge can be in matters of sex. When you are attempting to stimulate her G-spot and get her to ejaculate, you can expect one of the following responses.

Gushing Orgasm—You'll know it when you've almost drowned in it. This will generally not happen the very first time.

Slight Leakage—This is when a small amount of droplets will be expelled during orgasm. If you get these results early on, you can be sure gushing orgasms are in your near future.

Deeper Orgasm—Even if there is no fluid expelled, at the very least she will experience a deeper-than-normal orgasm.

"WTF"—This is when she gives you the "What the fuck do you think you're doing?" look because she is one of the very few women who doesn't respond to G-spot stimulation or you still don't know what the fuck you're doing!

If you get the second or third response from your partner, you can be pretty confident that you will soon know what it's like to make a woman gush. The G-spot can be trained, in a sense, along with the muscles that are involved in female ejaculation. The number of occasions the G-spot is stimulated and how strong the surrounding muscles become will be the factors that dictate the scope and intensity of her physical response, or, in other words, the amount of love juice she squirts in your face!

Sexercises for Her

There are exercises that women can do to target their "orgasm" muscles, and you're just the guy to show her how. Normally referred to as "Kegel exercises" (or pelvic floor exercises), these are very similar to the prostate exercises I described previously. This is the way I would go about introducing these exercises to her:

Talk to her about her "orgasm" muscles. Explain how they are used when she squeezes your penis during sex and that these are the same muscles she would use if somebody startled her while she was urinating and she cut off her urine flow midstream. Further explain how these muscles can actually be trained with specific exercises to become stronger and that stronger "orgasm" muscles will result in orgasms both more intense and easier to achieve, not to mention the increased ability to squeeze and tighten her vagina around your dingus. At this point, she should be sold!

Next, tell her the even better news that she can do these exercises anywhere and nobody will know she's doing them!

Look, if you're going to assume the role of personal pussy trainer you need to understand exactly what she needs to do and exactly why she

Kegel (pelvic floor) exercises derive their name from Dr. Arnold Kegel, a gynecologist who developed the exercises in 1948 as a method of controlling incontinence in women after childbirth. Dr. Kegel is also known for developing the Kegel perineometer, a device used for measuring vaginal pressure.

needs to do it that way. The first thing you need to do is help her identify her "orgasm" muscles, which are also called pelvic floor muscles. As I mentioned, these are the muscles she would use to stop her flow of urine. Some women will be weak in this area and find identifying and isolating these muscles difficult at first. Once you have helped her to understand the concept, showing her how to do the exercise should be a snap:

1. Identify the orgasm muscles
2. Isolate them by squeezing or pulling in and then releasing
3. Make sure the abdomen, thigh, and buttock muscles are relaxed and still while performing the exercise

After she is able to perform the exercise properly, it's time for her to adopt a sexercise regimen. Because there are two types of muscle fibers (fast-twitch and slow-twitch) being exercised, it is best to vary the speed of the squeezing. Take a look at the regimen below, as it includes the necessary variations:

Variation #1: Squeeze and hold for two seconds; repeat five to ten sets of twenty squeeze and holds
Variation #2: Squeeze and release immediately; repeat five to ten sets of twenty squeeze and releases
Variation #3: Squeeze and hold for ten seconds; repeat five to ten sets of twenty squeeze and holds

Just like any other exercise program, the number of repetitions performed should be incrementally increased as the muscles get stronger.

There are products available specifically designed to exercise these muscles. These include Kegel exercisers and weighted balls, usually two, some-times called ben wa balls. You can find out more about these types of products in chapter 27, but I do have to caution you about something based on a very embarrassing and dangerous personal experience . . .

It was the spring of 1999, and I was in Vegas with a girl I was dating named Malena. We were there for a getaway weekend of fun and fucking. After breakfast, we grabbed a cab to a nearby sex shop and loaded up on some goodies for later that evening. G-spot vibes, anal beads, lubricants, ben wa balls—I spent over three hundred bucks but I knew it would be worth every penny! Malena was a hottie but somewhat inexperienced. However, she was extremely open to trying new things. She had become pregnant by her high school sweetheart, they got married, she had the baby, he started cheating, and they got divorced—she hadn't heard from him in four years. Anyway, she had this thing about her pussy not being tight enough because she had a baby and she was really excited about the ben wa balls!

The plan for the evening was a nice dinner, followed by a Jacuzzi in the room and then some bada bing, if you know what I mean. Malena was looking good as we left the room—loose miniskirt, halter top, and five-inch heels. As we dropped from the twenty-third floor in a semicrowded elevator, Malena leaned into me and whispered, "I've got them inside of me now." I smiled but had no idea what she was talking about at first. Then she followed with, "You don't believe me?" and discreetly grabbed my hand and directed it to her pussy from behind. I probably figured it out before my hand actually reached her pussy but I stuck a finger inside to confirm—yup, she had the ben wa balls inside her all right, and she wasn't wearing panties either!

OK, fast-forward past an excellent dinner at a restaurant at our hotel. We were walking through the casino when I was approached by a very old friend and his wife. Neither of us had any idea the other was going to be in Vegas; they told us they had a table reserved at a nearby nightclub and invited us for a drink.

Now fast-forward about seventy-five minutes and two or three drinks each. Malena's favorite song started playing and she said we "have to" dance. There we were grooving on the dance floor when all of a sudden a ben wa ball shot from between Malena's legs, quickly followed by the

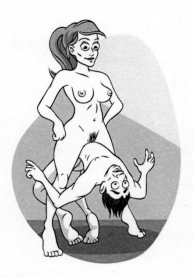

"OK, I take it back—your Kegel exercises
are definitely working."

other one. You should have seen the look on her face as they bounced a
few times, then started rolling across the dance floor. After her momentary shock, she quickly moved to start chasing one of them as it rolled toward the DJ booth. She attempted to use her foot to stop the rolling ball
by stepping on it as she ran after it, but this caused her to lose her balance
and fly backward, smashing the back of her head on the dance floor.
Thankfully, Malena and I were able to laugh about it later that night after
they finished stitching her head up and the pain medication set in. As a
matter of fact, laughing is about all we did the rest of our stay. Consider
yourself warned!

    To sum it all up, in my opinion the question as to whether or not fe-
male ejaculation exists should be grouped along with: "Does a bear shit in
the woods?" "Did Bush suck as a president?" and "Did O.J. do it?"—all of
which can be answered with a definite yes! Now let that soak in for a moment before we move on.

CHAPTER 18

Bun in the Oven

For a woman who engages in unprotected sex, her chances of becoming pregnant are always the same, approximately one out of twenty—even if it's her first time. A female can become pregnant any time after she begins to ovulate. This means that she could become pregnant even before she has her first period, since women start ovulating about fourteen days before their period begins. Here's how the whole pregnancy deal goes.

Females are born with about four hundred thousand eggs in their ovaries. Once females hit puberty they begin to ovulate. This is when, once each month, a few of those four hundred thousand eggs mature and one lucky devil is released from the ovary. While those eggs are maturing, the lining of the uterus becomes thicker to act as a protective shelter for the egg to implant in. If the egg is not fertilized with sperm within twelve to forty-eight hours of being released from the ovary, it will disintegrate. About two weeks later, the thick lining of the uterus is shed over a four-to-seven-day period of time—this is called menstruation and the entire process is known as the female reproductive cycle.

A female is most fertile when she is ovulating but can also become pregnant anywhere from five days before ovulation to one to two days afterward. These variations are mainly due to unknown "sperm survival" factors. That is, every guy's sperm has a different "shelf life" once it's been deposited into a vagina. Sperm can live inside the female body for up to five days!

The point is that every time you engage in unprotected vaginal sex it's a crapshoot. As a matter of fact, you've got better odds of getting a woman

Women who orgasm between one minute before and forty-five minutes after their partner's ejaculation retain 70 to 80 percent of his sperm. Women who orgasm more than one minute before their partner retain less than 50 percent of his sperm.

The sperm count of an average American male is down 30 percent from thirty years ago.

"For birth control, I rely on my personality."—Milt Abel

It takes sperm one hour to swim a distance of seven inches.

pregnant than you'll ever get in Vegas! Think about it next time you're considering "rolling the dice"!

Birth Control

In light of the above, it seems like the perfect time to talk about some of the birth control options you should be familiar with. Currently, there are over twenty-five different methods of birth control available to women and men. Here is a breakdown of the eleven most popular methods being used today.

Birth Control Effectiveness and Usage Chart

BIRTH CONTROL METHOD	TYPE OF CONTRACEPTION	EFFECTIVENESS RATE	PERCENTAGE OF TOTAL BIRTH CONTROL USED	COMMENTS
Pill	Hormonal	92 percent	31 percent	The pill would actually have a 99 percent effectiveness rate if women didn't forget to take it. Though considering some women have a tough time remembering to breathe, it's probably not the best choice for everyone.
Tubal Ligation	Sterilization	99 percent	27 percent	This is also referred to as a woman having her "tubes tied" and is a permanent birth control procedure that prevents pregnancy by preventing the egg from entering the uterus and blocks the passage of sperm up the fallopian tube.
Male Condom	Barrier	85 percent	18 percent	These have the added benefit of protecting against sexually transmitted disease. Also, when they are used in conjunction with a spermicide, their effectiveness rate jumps into the low 90 percent range. From a male perspective, the male condom, vasectomy, and the female condom, are the only methods you can really depend on, as they are the only ones you can see, feel, and control.

continued

BIRTH CONTROL METHOD	TYPE OF CONTRACEPTION	EFFECTIVENESS RATE	PERCENTAGE OF TOTAL BIRTH CONTROL USED	COMMENTS
Vasectomy	Sterilization	99 percent	9 percent	This is the male equivalent of tubal ligation, providing permanent birth control for men by preventing sperm from being transported out of the testes.
Depo-Provera Injection	Hormonal	97 percent	5 percent	This is a procedure in which a female is injected with the hormone progestin, which will prevent pregnancy for up to three months.
Withdrawal	Withdrawal	73 percent	4 percent	This is also referred to as "pulling out" and is the least effective of the methods mentioned. Issues like pre-come leakage and the man's timing and self-control play too much into the ultimate success or failure of the method for any couple to be able to count on it as a truly effective method of birth control.
Intrauterine Device (IUD)	Hormonal	99 percent	2 percent	A reversible method of birth control in which a small T-shaped device is inserted into the uterus to prevent pregnancy. Removal of the device will allow the female to become pregnant, under the right circumstances.

Here are four of the newer, more popular methods of birth control that have been gaining ground on the above methods.

BIRTH CONTROL METHOD	TYPE OF CONTRACEPTION	EFFECTIVENESS RATE	PERCENTAGE OF TOTAL BIRTH CONTROL USED	COMMENTS
Contraceptive Patch	Hormonal	98 percent	Unknown	This is an adhesive patch that is applied to a woman's skin, which slowly releases hormones through the skin and into the bloodstream.
Vaginal Ring	Hormonal	92 percent	Unknown	This is a device the female inserts in her vagina that slowly releases hormones that prevent pregnancy for a month.
Female Condom	Barrier	79 percent	Unknown	This is a polyurethane pouch with O-shaped rings on opposite ends. One ring sits around the closed end of the pouch and is inserted into the vagina. The other ring serves as the opening of the pouch and remains outside the vagina. At three bucks a pop, they're fairly pricey!
Essure	Sterilization	99 percent	Unknown	This is a newer type of sterilization process, meaning it's permanent, and it's unique because it requires no incisions to be made. It is a method in which tiny metal coils are inserted in a woman's fallopian tubes. Over time, scar tissue forms in and around the coils, which ultimately serves as a barricade, blocking the sperm from reaching the egg.

From my perspective, it is your responsibility to make sure you are having protected sex. I can't tell you how many times I've heard things like "But she told me she was on the pill!" or "She said she had her tubes tied!" or "I had no clue she had her IUD removed!"

The truth is, I've not only heard it from friends and acquaintances many times *but I've lived it!* It was a late February evening in 1996 and I had decided that my relationship with Tara was not working and I had to break it off. The conversation went almost exactly like this:

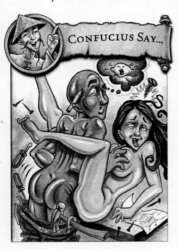

It takes many nails to build crib—but one screw to fill it

Me: Tara, I think we both realize this isn't working. I know it will take you some time to find a place but I want you to start looking now. I'll help in any way I can to get you in a place you're comfortable.

Tara: [with tears welling] I can't believe you're throwing a pregnant woman out on the street!

Me: Pregnant? What do you mean pregnant?

Tara: Oh, now you don't understand English? What kind of man would throw a pregnant woman out on the street?

Me: How could you be pregnant? You have that shit in your arm! [She was using a form of birth control called Norplant, a time-release device that is implanted in the upper arm.]

Tara: I suppose you're gonna say you don't remember me telling you that I had it removed because it was making me gain weight?

Me: *What? Are you fucking crazy?* You think I'd forget something like that?

Tara: Please stop yelling, you'll upset the baby.

I'm gonna stop there and spare you from the rest of the incredibly ridiculous details except to say that I was taught a very large lesson by that experience—unless you've had a vasectomy or are using some barrier method of protection that you can see and feel, you can't be 100 percent sure about anything!

By the way, eight months after that conversation, I stood in the delivery room and watched in amazement as my son made his grand entrance into the world while I simultaneously realized that my life would be forever changed from that moment on.

Urban Legend Recently Debunked

Using Coca-Cola as a douche after sex is not an effective method of birth control! I repeat, a Coca-Cola douche will not prevent pregnancy! According to the Boston University School of Medicine, while Coke was found to impede the mobility of sperm, it is not effective enough to keep the sperm from reaching the uterus. Now, if you're wondering what you should do with all that Coke you have in your cupboard, you could always drink it, or clean your car engine with it, or remove some rust with it, or you could always take small amounts of it and drip it onto your partner's pussy. Pour a small amount onto her clit and lap it up before it reaches her ass. The combined sensations that your tongue and the carbonation provide will be more than effective!

Can Anal Sex Lead to Pregnancy?

For those of you who know anything about me, it won't surprise you to know that anal sex is my preferred method of practicing birth control. Unfortunately, it's not 100 percent foolproof because there is a slight chance of the semen leaking from the anus after intercourse and dripping across the perineum or taint into the vagina. This is also known as a

If you have unprotected sex with the same chick for a year, there is an 85 percent chance that she will become pregnant during that time.

"splash conception." By the way, 8 percent of the couples who use anal sex as a method of birth control have babies each year. Personally, I enjoy anal sex so much, it's a risk I'm willing to take!

Condom Knowledge

If I had to choose one message for you to take from this book, it would have to be this—always use condoms with new partners. While it's probably the most unoriginal message in this book, it is also one of the most important! The consequences of having unprotected sex are far-reaching. Take a look at this chart to get a clear understanding of what I'm talking about.

The Pros and Cons of Wearing a Condom

PROS	CONS
Protects you from contracting HIV (this can kill you)	It feels slightly more pleasurable to have sex without one
Protects you from contracting herpes (there is no cure)	It makes having sex more expensive
Protects you from contracting syphilis (this causes blindness and death)	
Protects you from contracting gonorrhea (this is painful)	
Protects you from contracting chlamydia	
Protects a poor innocent baby from parents who aren't ready to be parents	
Protects your personal and financial future	

Those last two items in the pro column are references to unwanted pregnancies and the potential consequences that follow. Let's assume for a second that you get a woman pregnant the first time you have sex with her and she makes it clear that she wants to keep the baby—what does that mean to you? Well, unless you're ready to marry her, it could mean:

Not only was your penis engineered specifically for the purposes of impregnating women, it is also designed to foil other males from attempting to plant their seeds. The pronounced ridge of the head of your cock acts like a shovel of sorts as it will collect the invading semen on the "in-stroke" and expel it on the "out-stroke."

1. Having to pay a portion or all of her maternity expenses. These could include doctor visits, childbirth classes, and hospital costs.
2. Having to pay child support. The amount can vary greatly depending on each of your financial situations. However, just to give you an idea of some expenses associated with having a newborn in the US, take a look at these: diapers—$80–$90 per month; childcare—$700–$1,000 per month; formula—$70–$80 per month; baby clothing—$60–$80 per month; medical insurance for child—$150–$200 per month; and it will cost around $500 to set up the baby nursery. A lot will depend on where you live, as child support formulas vary from state to state.
3. Of course, you could opt for the shotgun wedding, which can seem like the easy way out. Beware, though, because it is most likely just a temporary solution to a long-term problem that could potentially add a heaping portion of "alimony al fresco" to your already overflowing plate.

Here are some other important things you should know about condoms:

Condoms are the most effective way to protect against STDs and unwanted pregnancies.

Latex and polyurethane condoms are the safest, most durable, and most widely available. Latex tends to be the more comfortable of the two because the material is more pliable than polyurethane.

It is possible for a man or a woman to have an allergic reaction to either latex or polyurethane. These reactions can include a

The first condom was invented in the 1500s and made of linen. Casanova used linen condoms.

painful rash but can be easily relieved by switching from latex to polyurethane or vice versa.

You should use only water-based or silicone-based lubricants with latex condoms. Oil-based lubricants can cause the latex to break down, causing tears or breaks.

You can use either water-based, silicone-based, or oil-based lubricants with polyurethane condoms. Polyurethane is a form of plastic and nothing breaks plastic down, except for certain types of alien blood.

Condoms should generally be stored in a cool, dry place. Don't store them in your wallet for extended periods of time as they can become damaged and worn out from the heat and pressure.

Make sure to squeeze any air bubbles out of the condom after you put it on to prevent the condom from bursting.

Placing one or two drops of lubricant into the tip of the condom before putting it on will add a level of comfort and increase the amount of sensation you feel.

Wearing two condoms at a time will not afford you any more protection and could actually cause both to tear because of friction between them.

There is no creative substitute for a condom. No matter how crazy it might seem, people have attempted do-it-yourself condoms using plastic sandwich bags, cling wrap, and even tinfoil. This is

"Condoms aren't completely safe. A friend of mine was wearing one and got hit by a bus."—Bob Rubin

not only completely stupid but could be extremely dangerous, too. Finally, whatever you do, don't follow the lead of Romanian Nicolae Popovici, who came up with what he thought was a "great idea" after his wife bought a batch of condoms that were a bit too large for him. Instead of buying some condoms that fit properly, Nicolae decided to superglue the oversized condom to his penis. Needless to say, Nicolae's ingenuity earned him a trip to the local hospital and, of course, the title of village idiot!

In summary . . .

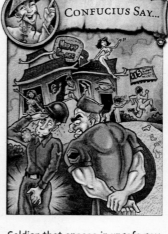

Soldier that engage in unsafe sex, risk dishonorable discharge

Always Use
Condoms
With New
Partners!

Conception Deception

Some of the stories I've heard about women using deceptive methods to get pregnant simply astound me! I'm amazed at the lack of consideration, toward both baby and partner, that behaviors like this convey. Women will usually cite one of two reasons for these "conception deceptions": their desire for the unconditional love of a baby, or their desire for the love of a particular man. The fact is, I can stand here on my soapbox and scream about it all day, but the bottom line is, there will always be certain women who will be willing to do anything to get pregnant, even if that means going to seemingly great lengths to achieve it! Take a gander at these tricks women use to get pregnant:

The Stop and Pop—This is when a woman will stop her birth control without her partner's knowledge. There's really not much a man can do about it either. I do recommend taking an obvious interest in the subject of birth control by initiating regular discussions about it. At the least, this could make her think twice about trying to deceive you in this way if she is so inclined.

The Sleeping Booty—Some women who are intent on getting pregnant will simply wait till you're sleeping or extremely inebriated to initiate sex

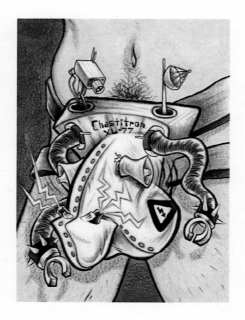

with you. This is a trick favored by women in relationships where condoms or pulling out are used as birth control methods. First, let me say if you're using the pull-out method you're already taking a huge risk. Anyway, the women who attempt this are counting on you not noticing that you're not wearing a condom or that you didn't pull out. Aside from never going to sleep or never getting drunk, I can't really offer a lot of advice on this one! It has got me thinking about some male chastity belt designs, though.

A fertility expert in Serbia claims to have developed a new method of birth control for men that is performed by delivering a low-voltage electric shock to the testicles. This is said to stun the man's sperm into a state of immobility for up to ten days.

The Sinking Ship—This should only be of concern to those of you using condoms in your relationship. All it takes is a pin or tack and some female ingenuity. A woman can simply prick a few tiny holes through a fully wrapped condom, knowing that it only takes a tiny amount of sperm to leak into her pussy for her to have a chance at becoming pregnant. Bringing your own condoms to each and every encounter will go a long way toward avoiding this type of deception.

The Pappy Smear—Have no doubt, a woman determined to get pregnant can be very resourceful. The pappy smear can be achieved in a number of different ways. It calls for the women to "come" into possession of the man's sperm and artificially inseminate herself with her fingers or some other tool her devious mind comes up with. Like I said, she can attain possession of your sperm in a number of different ways. She could give you a blow job and act like she swallowed, then excuse herself to go to the bathroom. When she is alone in the bathroom, she could spit some of the sperm she didn't swallow

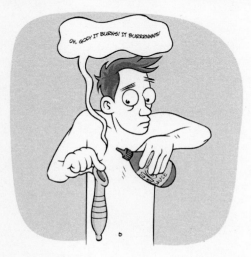

onto her fingers and then insert those fingers into her pussy, depositing the sperm as deep as she possibly can. Or she could retrieve your discarded condom from the trash and find a way to empty its contents into her pussy. Again, unless you have the intuition of a private dick, most men are defenseless against these kinds of tricks. I will mention, though, in regard to the discarded condoms, I have heard of one method of revenge that has been implemented with success by some men who suspected their partners of pappy smearing: slyly putting a tiny amount of hot sauce in their discarded condoms.

How Paternity Testing Works

Paternity testing is the basic term used for tests to determine who is the father of a child. It is performed by collecting DNA samples from the child and suspected father. This is usually done by taking saliva samples from the insides of their cheeks. The samples are then sent off to a paternity testing laboratory, where they are analyzed to establish a DNA profile for each individual involved. These profiles are then examined to see if there are enough similarities (matching DNA markers) in the DNA profiles of the child and suspected father to establish clear paternity. This method of establishing paternity is considered 99.9 percent reliable and can usually be completed within a three-or-four-day period. In the case of disputed paternity before the child has been born, there is a type of test called a prenatal paternity test, but it must be approved by a doctor and does pose a small risk to the unborn child.

There are home paternity-testing kits available for purchase. While they can be used only to establish the paternity of a child already born, they are considered to be 99.9 percent reliable. However, you should know that in order for a paternity test to be admissible in court, you must have it performed in a doctor's office.

Sex During Pregnancy

If your partner is experiencing a normal pregnancy, sex is considered safe during all stages of the pregnancy. Many men worry that they will harm the baby with their penis (maybe poke its eye out?) or by causing their partner to orgasm. The fact is your baby is well protected by the amniotic sac and the strong muscles of the uterus. There are some positions that work better for sex during pregnancy, especially as your partner gets further along and her belly gets bigger.

Kneeling/Standing Missionary—Your partner should lie on her back with her knees drawn into her chest or legs extending over your shoulders. If she is lying in the middle of the bed, you would kneel in front of her. If she is on the edge of the bed you can stand in front of her. Placing a pillow under her tushy in either scenario will make her more comfortable.

Spoon—Your partner should lie on her side and curl up in a C shape as you lie on your side behind her.

During World War II, condoms were used to cover rifle barrels to keep them from being damaged by saltwater as soldiers swam to shore.

"We all worry about the population explosion, but we don't worry about it at the right time."—Arthur Hoppe

There are some who feel it is so important for you to use condoms, they are willing to give them to you at no charge. Check out Getfreecondoms.org for more info.

From Behind—Your partner would either get on all fours with her head down on the bed or bent over the bed (or whatever), with you entering from behind while kneeling or standing.

Woman on Top—This one is pretty self-explanatory. The benefit of this, as well as the other positions I've discussed, is it aims to help you avoid one thing—placing weight or direct pressure on your pregnant partner's belly.

There is one thing you should never, ever do while having sex with a pregnant woman—blow directly into her pussy! This can cause an air embolism, which can be potentially fatal to both child and mother.

BOOK III

ABOUT SEX

CHAPTER 19

Foreplay Gets You More Play

Expecting a woman to have sex without any foreplay is like a coach asking an athlete to take the field without warming up. It's stupid! Considering foreplay can be as light as a massage or as effortless as some passionate kissing, the man who ignores foreplay either doesn't care or just doesn't get it.

Of course, foreplay doesn't end at massage or kissing, nor does it begin there. Foreplay is about setting the mood, and this can start with paying attention to details, like making sure your sheets are clean, setting the proper lighting, playing the right music, and making sure the room is cozy and warm. Foreplay is the time to talk, learn, tease, have fun, and explore.

I do understand that for whatever reason, it is difficult for many of you to express yourselves or even associate the idea of teasing or having fun with sex. Trust me when I say you have so much more to gain by adapting these types of attitudes toward sex than you have to lose. With that in mind, below you will find a few activities you should consider incorporating into your foreplay sessions:

Get Her Wet—Draw her a warm bath and set her up with a romance novel. In addition to the fact that she will love you doing this for her, the warm water will help her relax and stimulate blood flow. If you want to get fancy you could add bubbles or specially formulated bath concoctions like Dr. Teal's Vapor Bath, which Mirna happens to be especially fond of. A variation on this would be to simply place a towel soaked in almost-hot

EROGENOUS ZONES

*(The areas on her body most sensitive
to sexual stimuli)*

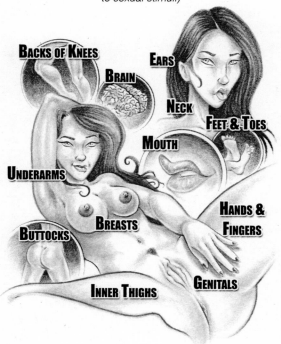

BACKS OF KNEES

BRAIN

EARS

NECK

FEET & TOES

MOUTH

UNDERARMS

HANDS & FINGERS

BREASTS

BUTTOCKS

GENITALS

INNER THIGHS

water directly over her pussy. Leave in place for a period of three to four minutes while you keep her busy by kissing her, fondling her, and occasionally giving her pussy a light slap through the towel. The heat from the towel will help to expand her blood vessels, which in turn will increase blood flow into her genital area, making her more sensitive and more easily stimulated.

Water Worx—You could also jump into that bathtub with her. Position yourself behind her, your chest against her back with your legs extended along the outside of hers. Turn the faucet on to flow a light stream of warm water. Guide her to lean back into your body as she draws her knees up toward her shoulders until her pussy is floating just above the water

Just to save you poets some time, there are no words in the dictionary that rhyme with "purple," "orange," or "silver."

line. Now gently position her so the water drops directly onto her hot box. You can vary the pressure of the water flow to increase or decrease stimulation and adjust the temperature to her liking. Since you're supporting her with your torso, your hands will be free to play with her tits or spank her inner thighs—whatever you think will float her boat.

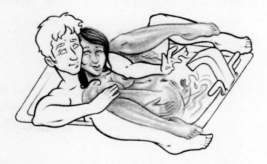

Sexy Texts—Send her a naughty text message during the day telling her some of the things you are going to do to her later that night. The anticipation of it all will have her literally marinating in her own juices all day as she watches the clock and thinks about what awaits her when she gets home! Here are a few examples of the type of text message I might send to Mirna. Obviously, she is not overly sensitive to or easily offended by the language I choose to use. Having said that, choose your words carefully, as you could easily turn a woman off by being too aggressive or using crude expressions.

1. You are invited for a night on the town
   lots of drinking and dancing
   before we get down!

2. I'll pick you up at eight
   and take you out to dine
   then back to my place
   for some hot 69!

3. Lips so soft
   body so tight
   can't wait to see you
   gonna fuck you all night!

Of course, poetry is not necessary but I guarantee you she will appreciate the creative, personal touch!

Mutual Masturbation—Put on her favorite X-rated movie, then each of you lie back, relax, and start masturbating. Many people cringe at the thought of others even knowing they masturbate, let alone doing it in front of someone. Many couples can spend a lifetime together (at least it seems like a lifetime for some couples) and never see each other masturbate. Doing it together, at the same time, is a way to even the playing field or decrease the embarrassment factor. Sharing this type of experience together will only strengthen the bond between you and lay the groundwork for further sexual exploration. Plus, an observant man can learn a lot about how and where a woman likes to be touched just by watching her masturbate—and vice versa, of course!

Role-Playing—There's something about assuming an alternate character or persona that allows people to open their minds to things they might not have considered before. Role-playing tends to blur the line between reality and fantasy, which makes for an atmosphere very conducive to sexual exploration. For many of you, this type of sex play seems like a waste of time, but it won't to her! I promise you she will appreciate the effort you make. I'm guessing your next question is "How would I go about initiating something like this?" I know this is going to sound like a strange answer, but you could talk to her about it, or if that sounds like too direct an approach to handle, you could send her a note, text, or e-mail like this:

Doctor/Patient Scenario

"This is a courtesy reminder that you have an appointment with Dr. Feelgood at ten P.M. tonight."

Or

"My girlfriend, she's like: 'What about foreplay?' I go: 'Honey, didn't I slap you around already today?'"—Andrew Dice Clay

Master/Slave Scenario

"Master Dick has heard you've been a very naughty girl today! He hereby demands your presence in his chambers at exactly eleven P.M. tonight to discuss your appropriate punishment."

Here are some other role-playing scenarios that you might be interested in exploring:

Stripper/client scenario
Hooker/client scenario
Maid/employer scenario
Artist/model scenario
Delivery boy/housewife scenario

If role-playing is something that sounds interesting, you should visit Roleplayingfantasies.com. Not only do they have a great selection of role-playing costumes, they also carry a wide variety of role-playing scripts for those of you who are less creatively inclined.

Be a Teacher

Any time you are able to teach a woman something new you will gain an added measure of respect and admiration from her. As a matter of fact, I'm willing to wager that by the time you've finished this book you'll be able to teach any woman you have intimate contact with something new. That is, unless you happen to be dating Madonna, Cher, Dr. Ruth, Lindsay Lohan, Tila Tequila, Paris Hilton, Pam Anderson, a porn star, or one of the girls from the Bunny Ranch, in which case—all bets are off! Now, if that "something new" you happen to teach her also adds to your sexual experience, all the better. My original intention here was to lay out a step-by-step guide to teach your partner how to give you what the Eskimos called a "blotla," or as I would very roughly translate, an "Eskimo mind-blower." Then I realized that since this requires your partner to have her mouth full of walrus blubber while she blows you and stick a frozen herring up your ass when you're just about to come, it was not going to be a viable option for many of you. Instead I'm going to delve into the art of deep throating and share with you some tips I have observed and learned from some of the greatest oral artists to ever live.

Teach Her How to Deep Throat—Like sushi, deep throating is an acquired taste for many women and if it doesn't go down right, a very messy situation could ensue. It is also a skill and for some enthusiasts even an art that when performed properly can be extremely satisfying for both the giver and receiver. Aside from the desire to swallow a penis, all deep throaters have one thing in common—control of their gag reflexes. This is the key to deep throating. Once you can help her master this, the rest will come easy for her . . . and so will you!

Controlling Her Gag Reflex—The fact is, most women who can deep throat learned the trick simply by practicing with a dick. As with any skill, practice makes perfect and deep throating is no exception. Here you would instruct your partner to take your cock in her mouth to the point that she feels her gag reflex start to respond and hold it there for a period of ten seconds. Once she is comfortable with your dipstick at that depth, she would take it a half inch deeper and hold until she again feels she has her gag reflex under control at this depth. This should be repeated until she is able to swallow your cock completely. The entire process could take days or weeks, depending on the woman. Of course, as I mentioned earlier, this method of practicing on you could get messy. Trust me on this; I speak from multiple experiences, however the first was the worst and most memorable. Sophia and I were in the front seat of my green Cadillac, which was parked in front of her apartment building in Hollywood. It was approaching midnight on a Friday, getting dangerously close to Sophia's curfew. Earlier in the day, I had picked Sophia up from Immaculate Conception, an all-girl Catholic school, and taken her down to Hollywood Boulevard to catch a movie and eat some dinner at the same place we had gone on our first date almost four months prior. By now, less than 120 days into our relationship, we were both convinced it was love . . . but we hadn't had sex yet. Sure I was finger-banging her and she had given me a few hand jobs, but that had been the extent of it. You see, Sophia was a virgin. It was important to her that she waited for the "right person" and for it to happen at the "right moment." Her mother was adamant that Sophia waited until she was married and she wasn't afraid to express it to either of us. She wasn't afraid of much actually. She stood at an even five feet and had to weigh in at a minimum of 280 pounds. She had an extremely sharp tongue, a mean left-hook, and surprisingly nimble feet. I often wondered how that woman gave birth to the five foot six, 115-pound blond-haired blue-eyed perfectly proportioned piece of ass that I called "honeybuns". . . but never out loud!

So there we sat in my green Cadillac. We had been making out for the last ten minutes or so when Sophia gently pushed away from me, unbuttoned and unzipped my jeans and pulled them down to my ankles. Then she reached her hand through the "piss slot" in my boxers and started playing with my boner. . . .

Sophia: I want to give you a blowjob.
Me: Really?
Sophia: Yeah, but you have to tell me if I'm doing it wrong.
Me: [laughing] I don't think there is a wrong way to give a blow job.
Sophia: That's not true! Brent still makes fun of Karen for leaving teeth marks on his dick. She made him bleed . . . how embarrassing.
Me: Okay, I promise to tell you if you're doing it wrong.
Sophia: Promise?
Me: Promise!

Sophia moved in to kiss me, hand still on boner, then slowly began working her mouth south. Her mouth was large enough to accommodate her own fist (a feat I had witnessed on numerous occasions and one of the reasons I had such confidence in her oral abilities), and was rimmed with naturally thick, luscious lips. I was not disappointed when she finally wrapped them around my penis like a velvet-lined glove and I made sure to let her know it. The more I made my pleasure known, the more exaggerated and enthusiastic her oral antics became. Soon she was pushing my cock against the back of her throat and I heard her gag and then . . . SPLAT! My lap looked like a Vegas buffet for babies featuring clam chowder, pureed chicken picatta, and the cream of crème brûlée. I could see a frightened look in Sophia's eyes as she lifted her head:

Sophia: Oh my God . . . I can't believe I just did that! I'm so sorry.
Me: [staying cool] Hey, don't worry and don't apologize. It's not like you did it on purpose. Can you do me a favor though and reach into the backseat and grab that towel?

Just as Sophia grabbed hold of the towel, there was a loud knocking on the passenger window. It startled the shit out of both of us. That's when I noticed the car windows were completely fogged up. So much so we could only see a light shadow of the fist hitting the window. Then we heard a familiar voice bellow, "Sophia, are you in there? Sophia, what are you doing in there? What are you doing to my daughter?"

Sophia: [whispering] Oh my God . . . it's my mother! What should we do?
Me: [whispering] Tell her you'll be out in a minute.
Sophia: [loud] Mom, I'll be right out.
Mom: What are you doing in there? Open the door.
Sophia: [loud] We're just talking. Go back inside and I'll be out in a minute.
Mom: Why can't you open the door? Are you naked? What is that animal doing to you?
Me: [whispering] Tell her we had a fight and we'll be finished talking in five minutes.
Sophia: [loud] Mom, we had a big fight and we're just talking. Please go back inside and I'll be right in.
Mom: Okay, if you're not inside within five minutes I'm gonna ground you for the next month.

And then there was silence. We waited two to three minutes before Sophia cleared a small spot of our heavy breath off the window and declared the coast clear with a sigh of relief. She helped me with the cleanup, we took a moment to gather ourselves and we exited the car. Instead of walking her to the door of her apartment as I normally would, this time I stopped about twenty feet short and gave her a good-night kiss. I didn't want to risk being subjected to a midnight interrogation by Sophia's mom. Once I saw her walk through the doorway, I turned to leave when I heard Sophia yell out, "Adam, wait." She ran up to me and said, "My mom has some chocolate chip cookies she wants to give you to take home. She seems fine. Come in for a minute. She makes really good cookies!" So I went into the apartment with Sophia, who led me into the kitchen where her mom stood holding a baking sheet full of chocolate chip cookies. Sophia's mom smiled when she saw me and said, "Go ahead, taste one and then I'll pack the rest of these up for you." I grabbed one off the sheet and said "Thank you" before taking a bite. Sophia was right, that was a good cookie. I was about to verbalize something to that effect, but before I could spit the words out, I stood like a deer caught in headlights as I watched Sophia's mom quickly raise the cookie sheet above her head then just as quickly slam it down on mine. Cookies flew everywhere!

Me: Ouch! Jesus Christ, what are you doing?

Mom: What were you trying to do with my daughter? [Then she hit me over the head a second time.] And don't take the Lord's name in vain!

Me: Ouch! I wasn't trying to do anything. We had a fight and we were talking.

Sophia: Mom, are you crazy? [Then turning to me.] Oh my God . . . are you all right?

Me: Yeah, I'm okay but I should probably go now.

On that sour note I left, jumped in my Caddy, and drove off wondering what would become of me and "honeybuns." I took Sunset Boulevard. I liked driving Sunset, especially on weekend nights when the streets were being cruised by the coolest, most expensive whips and the sidewalks spilled over with VIPs and wannabees . . . and hookers. So, I'm driving down Sunset and I caught glimpse of a tall blond girl in a very short, bright blue miniskirt standing on a street corner. Coincidentally, it was at that exact moment that I was struck again—this time by the fact that I didn't get off earlier with Sophia and that I was extremely horny. Suddenly, as if someone had flipped on my autopilot switch, I found myself making a right turn. And then another one. And then another until I magically arrived at the same street corner as the tall blonde. She was puffing on a cigarette now. I noticed she was a bit larger than she seemed at first glimpse, but I smiled anyway. She approached my car and leaned into the passenger side window.

Tall Blonde: [in a raspy voice that I attributed to the cigarettes] Hi, honey, you looking for a date?
Me: I am.
Tall Blonde: Are you a cop?
Me: No. Are you a cop?
Tall Blonde: You ever seen any cops that look like this, honey?

Then she jumped into the passenger seat and told me to drive up the street (which I did) and that she would tell me where to park (which she did).

Tall Blonde: Okay, now honey, how much money you got?
Me: I just want a blowjob. How much for that?
Tall Blonde: You got twenty bucks?
Me: Yeah.
Tall Blonde: All right then, take down your pants.

I started to unbutton my jeans. It was exactly that moment that I remembered the reason I had not gotten off with Sophia . . . she had puked all over my cock! And now I have just asked this stranger to put it in her mouth. I quickly rebuttoned my pants.

Me: Oh, shit! I didn't realize how late it is. I can't do this now. I'm sorry. I'll come back some other time.
Tall Blonde: Relax, honey. Trust me, this won't [reaching for my jeans] take long.

Me: [pushing her hand away] No, really I can't do this now.

Tall Blonde: Look asshole, I don't know what kind of game you're trying to play, but I want my money.

Me: [reaching into my back pocket for wallet] Fine. Here's your twenty dollars.

As I looked up from my wallet to hand her the money, I saw a small handgun pointed at my face.

Me: What the fuck are you doing?

Tall Blonde: I don't like games. Give me all your money, the chain, and your watch.

I gave her everything I had.

Tall Blonde: Don't go to the cops or my man will hunt you down and kill you!

Then she was gone and I was left to contemplate the evening's events during what seemed like an unusually long drive home that Friday night. Did I report it to the police? Hell no! Though, it may interest you to know that while we never married, my relationship with Sophia survived that night and she eventually found me to be that "right person" to share her most guarded possession with. I have no idea what Sophia really thinks about that decision she made, but I can tell you with absolute certainty that her mom wasn't happy about it!

So, as I was saying, letting her practice with your penis can have its drawbacks. Which brings me to another method of gaining control of the gag reflex. This calls for her to use her toothbrush to brush her tongue on the spot where her gag reflex begins. She should brush this area for a period of eight to ten unpleasant seconds, as she will most likely be gagging the duration. This process should be repeated over the next couple of days until she is actually able to touch that spot with her toothbrush without gagging. Now it would be time to move the toothbrush slightly farther back on the tongue to the new spot where her gag reflex begins and to repeat the daily brushing process. As she continues to get comfortable at each new "spot," she should continue to move the brushing area farther back on her tongue until she feels she has gained control over her gag reflex. No matter which method or combination of methods is used, the ability to control her gag reflex will not instantly transform her into a "deep throat artiste." There are a few other things she should know:

Lubricating Her Throat—There are two ways to achieve this. One is when you stick a funnel in her mouth and squeeze a tube of KY Jelly down her gullet . . . no, no, no I'm just joking, but I do know of some women who take so much pride in their deep throat skills that they swallow a teaspoon of olive oil beforehand. I personally have had the pleasure of experiencing a well-oiled esophagus on a few occasions and highly recommend it. The other way would be for her to learn how to produce the required lubrication naturally. She can do this by taking your cock in her mouth, pressing its tip against the back of her throat and either holding it there for ten seconds or gently tapping it against the back of her throat using short head bobs, for the same period of time. Gagging at this time will actually help her to produce the thick, stringy, slick saliva that will coat her throat and make your knockwurst that much easier for her to swallow.

Expanding Her Throat—If she pulls her tongue down and back toward her throat, this will help to make her throat more spacious and accommodating for your penis.

Staying Relaxed—The more relaxed her mind and throat is the better. Consistently breathing in through her mouth and out through her nose will help her to get and stay relaxed.

Remember, this is not something that a woman is going to learn to perfect overnight. It will take desire and effort on her part in combination with patience and support from you . . . the type of collaboration that deep throat dreams are made of.

Here's one more mutually satisfying trick to mystify her with:

Tighten the Screw—Women will do vaginal exercises and some even resort to surgical procedures in their quest for a tighter pussy. Neither of which, by the way, am I discouraging. The fact is that a tighter pussy does equate to more pleasurable sex for both participants. Instead I'm going to tell you about a "quick fix," so to speak. Something you can show her that will make her wonder, "How the fuck does he know that?" Here's what you do: Before having sex, empty the solution out of a douche container and fill it with 4½ ounces of warm water. Add ½ teaspoon of aluminum sulfate to the water, mix thoroughly, and have her douche with it as she would normally. The aluminum will cause the inner walls of her vagina to contract around your penis. This same formula can be used as an enema for you anal enthusiasts. No matter the orifice you fancy, this little trick will give new meaning to the word "squeezebox" for you and have her feeling like a near-virgin again.

The truth is foreplay can be many things to many people. There is no set of rules to operate by. Hell, in my current relationship, we consider everything but anal sex to be foreplay! The bottom line is that a man will never be considered a great lover by women unless he has mastered the art of foreplay—the art of making his partner feel wanted, appreciated, beautiful, sexy, and ready for anything!

Before we move on, I want to mention another opportunity afforded by the concept of foreplay: the opportunity to inconspicuously inspect the genitals of a new partner.

Clam Exam—This is a technique for doing a covert visual inspection of your prospective partner's genital area for signs of STDs. Here's how it works:

Once you've removed all her clothes, place a pillow under her pelvis as you lay her facedown. You've now got her in a fantastic position to give her an ass massage. Besides the fact that women love to have their asses fondled and squeezed, having her in this position will give you the chance to do a thorough visual inspection of her genital area.

About 1 percent of women can orgasm solely from breast stimulation.

"I think you're running into a lot of trouble if your idea of foreplay is, 'Brace yourself, honey, here I come!'"—Phil McGraw

CHAPTER 20

The Cunning Linguist

There are two kinds of pussy eaters out there: those who do it because they feel they have to, and those who do it because they want to. Let's be honest, some of you guys approach pussy like a starving Indian would a tandoori chicken, while others go at it like it's a cod liver oil lollipop.

This is where the men are separated from the boys when it comes to eating pussy. Men want to do it, and boys do it because they feel they have to. And believe me when I tell you women are experts at telling the men from the boys.

I love eating pussy. I get off on the idea of pleasuring a woman, of having that kind of power—the power to drive her absolutely crazy with ecstasy. In a somewhat selfish way, I am also motivated by knowing that there is a very good chance that my effort will not only be appreciated but reciprocated . . . and then some.

The bottom line is no matter which category you fall into, I'm about to lay out some great pussy-eating tips and techniques.

If you're in the group that does it because they like it, well, you're on your way to becoming a master cunnilinguist. The rest of you should take some acting classes after you're finished with this book, because no matter your skill or technique, if your heart's not into it, she'll know it!

Before I get into specific techniques, I want to touch on a few general yet very important facts and rules.

The Clitoris—There are three parts to a woman's clitoris: the glans, the shaft, and the hood. You will find that all women are different in regard to the size of their clit and the size and tightness of their hood. The hood serves as protection for the shaft and glans, much like the foreskin of an uncircumcised penis. While most women find both pleasurable, it is a different sensation when their clits are licked/sucked with the hood intact as opposed to the hood being pulled back and the glans being fully exposed. Generally, you want to pull the hood back when you're really digging in and trying to get her off.

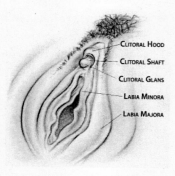

CLITORAL HOOD
CLITORAL SHAFT
CLITORAL GLANS
LABIA MINORA
LABIA MAJORA

Pressure/Force—You must always remember that every woman will have a different threshold for how much pressure you apply to her clit, how much force you use with your fingers, and how many fingers you place inside her pussy or ass. I have always found it best to start slow and light and let the woman dictate the pace.

Talking/Making Noise—Women want to know what you're thinking and that you're enjoying what you're doing. Don't be afraid to pay a compliment or two to your partner's vagina. I know this type of verbalization is more difficult for some of you than others, but just think about how reassuring a few complimentary words could be to a woman. Keep in mind that most women grow up with the notion that their vagina is unattractive, especially when compared to other women's. It really doesn't take a lot of effort and could be as simple as:

You looking at her pussy and telling her how beautiful it is

or

You saying, "What a pretty pussy," as you remove her panties

or

You whispering in her ear, "I can't wait to taste your pussy!"

or

After the first few licks, you say, "If this is all-you-can-eat, I'm gonna be here for a while!"

Aside from being complimentary, women prefer noisy eaters. I didn't say sloppy eaters, I said noisy. I'm referring to sounds of appreciation—that's the way women see it at least. Imagine what a world-class chef would feel like if he served up his signature dish and stood by waiting for the diner's approval, but the diner ate the meal in complete silence. That chef would immediately begin to wonder if the diner liked what he was served. Well, women are like chefs; they want to know you're enjoying your meal. This one's even easier than the compliments—all you need to do is start practicing by putting your lips against the back of your hand and singing the first three words of the Campbell's Soup song (mmm, mmm, good) without removing your lips from your hand. Seriously though, silence is not golden when it comes to eating pussy.

Teasing—You should never start in on the pussy without a bit of teasing to get her going. Just as important, however, the teasing shouldn't stop just because the pussy eating has started. You have absolutely nothing to lose by sprinkling in a dash of tease throughout the entire oral encounter.

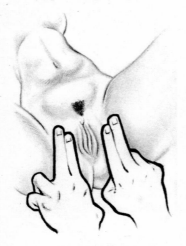

Pussy Massage

There are many ways to go about teasing a woman, but for the sake of time and space, I will only go into a few of my favorites.

Kissing/Licking—I'm mainly referring to kissing and licking the parts of her body that surround her genital area, including stomach, hips, inner thighs, pubic mound, ass cheeks, taint, and asshole.

Massage—Also a great way to tease. Her inner thighs, lower back, and ass are prime targets, but if you really want to get her juices flowing, try gently massaging her labia majora and pubic mound.

Pussy Pinching—This is a lighter, more seductive form of pinching. It is done by placing your hand over her vagina and grabbing the folds of skin between your fingers. This technique allows you to stimulate her

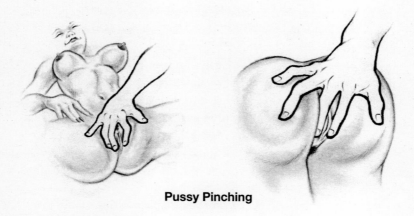

Pussy Pinching

clit by manipulating (squeezing, pulling, and using a gentle up/down motion) the folds of her skin to create friction or pressure.

Pussy Slap—A few gentle, well-placed slaps to her clitoris and labia will be certain to get her attention. You'll instantly know if she likes it and she'll tell you if she wants you to slap harder.

Oral Techniques

Here are twelve surefire oral techniques for you to experiment with on your partner(s):

1. **Flick**—You quickly and repeatedly use the tip of your tongue to flick her clit.
2. **Stroke**—This calls for you to extend and flatten out your tongue as you repeatedly brush it over her love button.
3. **Slap**—Same as above except you gently slap at her clit with your flattened tongue.
4. **Suck**—Place your lips over her clitoris and use a gentle suction while running your tongue over it at the same time. This is also very effective to use on her labia majora and minora. Again, start with light pressure and let her dictate the rest.

Another variation would be to place your lips over her hood and glans and gently suck the hood back and forth over the glans.

5. **Blowing**—Lightly blowing on her wet pussy and clit will cause a different kind of sensation and stimulation for her. Whatever you do, *don't* blow directly *into* her pussy.

6. **Humming**—Humming while gently holding her clit between your lips can be very stimulating to your partner. Placing your entire mouth over her pussy and humming while flicking her clit with your tongue as she is about to come can produce mind-blowing results.

7. **Raspberries**—You know how you simulate farting sounds by putting your lips and tongue against a body part and blowing? Well, do it on her clitoris and see how she reacts. Again, never blow directly into her vagina.

8. **Alphabet**—The late comedian Sam Kinison made this technique famous by referencing it in one of his routines: Use your tongue to trace the letters of the alphabet over her pleasure peanut. The technique itself is no joke, however, and can be extremely enjoyable for your partner, along with giving those of you with ADD something to help you maintain your focus!

9. **Figure Eights**—Using your tongue, you trace the outline of the number eight as small (concentrating on her clitoris) or as large (from her love button down to her butthole) as you or she likes.

10. **Probe**—Here you take your tongue and dip it in and out of her love canal.

11. **Grinder**—Extend and flatten your tongue and grab hold of your partner's hips while encouraging her to grind her pussy against your tongue. She can hold on to the sides of your head to gain added leverage.

12. **Double Dip**—Appropriately, there are two ways to execute the double dip. You can either position yourself with your tongue in her ass and your nose in her pussy or position yourself with your tongue in her pussy and your nose in her ass.

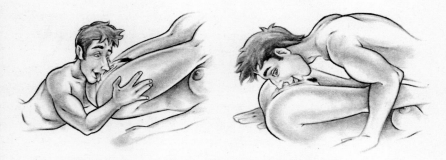

This is definitely an advanced maneuver but it's sure to be appreciated by anally inclined women.

Tongue Patterns

These are patterns that you trace along her body with your tongue. A cunning linguist will know the following patterns or routes like the back of his own hand:

The Figure 8—See page 188.

The Alphabet—See page 188.

The Happy Trail—Run your tongue from her belly button to her love button.

The End Around—Run your tongue from her clitoris to her butt-hole, circle it a few times, then run it back up to her clitoris.

The Home Run—Imagine superimposing a baseball infield over her vagina. It would look something like this:

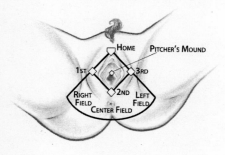

Now, use your tongue to circle the bases as you take multiple home run trots. In this scenario, or a similar one, you can really let go and get creative. Have fun with it . . . add some play-by-play shtick, for example:

You: Before we get to the first pitch, please join us in humming our national anthem.

Action: You hum the national anthem on her bliss berry.

You: The pitcher has finished warm-ups and looks at the catcher. He shakes off the first sign . . .

Action: Wiggle your tongue at her vaginal entrance.

You: Now he goes into his windup . . . and here's the pitch!

Action: Quick circular motions around her vaginal entrance, then her clit.

You: He swings . . .

Action: Flick her clit.

You: Oh my! It's a long drive to center field . . .

Action: Run tongue from clit to asshole.

You: He hit it deep . . .

Action: Stick your tongue deep in her pussy or ass (whichever she'll appreciate more).

You: It's going . . .

Action: Circle bases with your tongue a few times.

You: It's going . . .

Action: Circle bases with your tongue a few more times.

You: It's gone! And the crowd goes crazy . . .

Action: Lay a bunch of raspberries all over her infield.

Yeah, it might sound corny, but this is the kind of stuff that helps create a fun, relaxed atmosphere in your bedroom!

Women who went to college are more likely to enjoy both giving and receiving oral sex than high-school dropouts.

"I have never been with a man who has performed any kind of good cunnilingus. Guys always act really bored. It's like they're . . . doing you a favor."—Jennifer Tilly

More Fun and Games

Sex Spells—Blindfold your partner, then use your tongue on her vagina or clitoris to trace the letters of a word and see if she can guess what you are spelling.

Great Positions for Cunning Linguists

69—This is a great position not only for mutual satisfaction but also for using fingers or toys on her. Keep in mind, there are some women who won't be able to orgasm in this position because they find having a cock and balls in their face to be somewhat distracting. In that case I recommend you try . . .

68—In this position, the man is on top with his arms straddling his partner's thighs. However, instead of straddling her head with his knees, he keeps both knees to one side of her head. Here you get the same great access as in 69, but without the distraction factor. Of course, she'll owe you one when you're done.

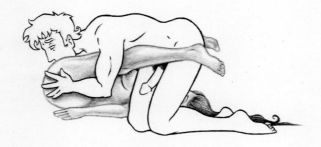

"Anyone can be passionate, but it takes real lovers to be silly."
—Rose Franken

Missionary—Allows for total access to both her pussy and ass, plus it is perfect for eye contact!

Close Shave—Lie flat on your back and have your partner straddle your face while on her knees. Make sure that she is facing you for eye contact purposes. Now grab hold of her hips and encourage her to grind herself on your lips and tongue. It makes for a nice change-up to put her in control of the pace and friction levels. I call it the close shave because this one could be painful for her if you aren't clean-shaven.

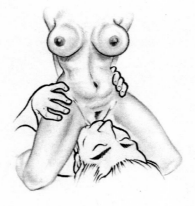

CHAPTER 21

The Motion of the Ocean

disagree with the "bigger is better" myth; I am a big believer in the adage "It's not the size of the boat but the motion of the ocean." To say it again, the size of your cock has nothing to do with whether or not your partner considers you a great lover. It's what you do with it that makes all the difference. Luckily for you, that is exactly what I'm going to focus on here. Before I go into specifics, I do want you to consider one thing: No matter how many suggestions I give you, it is incumbent upon you to know when to pull them out of your new bag of tricks. So much of sex is about intuition. Knowing when to do something is just as important as knowing what to do. Unfortunately, intuition is not something that can be taught. It comes down to a combination of how intimately you know your partner and simply trusting your instincts. Now, let's take a look at some of the different types of penile thrusting techniques you can use during vaginal or anal intercourse:

1. **The Slow Jam**—I mention this one first because it's not so much about thrusting technique as it is about how you initially insert your penis into your partner. It is simply a matter of inserting the tip of your penis inside your partner and ever so slowly working it in with a series of short, measured strokes that you very gradually allow to get deeper and deeper until you achieve maximum penetration. If you do it right, you'll have to stop her from trying to pull you all the way inside her, as the anticipation will drive her nuts!

2. **The Longfellow**—This is where you insert yourself to maximum

depth and pull out as far as possible without popping out, with long, measured strokes. This is a technique that provides maximum penetration and stimulation for your partner. Used in the right positions, it is also an excellent technique to use to stimulate her G-spot. The head of your penis will inevitably come into contact with it as it thrusts along the entire length of her love tunnel.

3. **The Merry-Go-Round**—This is where you thrust with circular motions, enabling you to hit all four walls of her pussy or ass. Varying the motion with full and half circles, switching up between clockwise and counterclockwise directional paths, and varying the depth of your thrusts provide you with plenty of opportunity to pump loads of motion into her ocean!

4. **The Hip-Hop**—This is a technique that entails you bouncing or hop-thrusting from side to side while inside of her. It is really only effective in two specific positions—the woman on her back with her legs thrown over the man's shoulders, or doggie style, with the man in the up-and-over position—but effective it is. Obviously, the bouncing action here is going to result in maximum penetration.

5. **The Shortstop**—Here you withdraw your penis almost entirely and start using a series of measured one-to-two-inch thrusts. This should put your penis at perfect G-spot depth.

6. **The Deep Six**—The exact opposite of the Shortstop. This technique calls for you to achieve maximum depth of penetration, retreating one to two inches and thrusting back to maximum depth. I have found these quick, short, deep strokes to be very popular with my partners.

7. **The Daily Grind**—A variation on the Deep Six, this one calls for you to again attain maximum depth, only this time you're going to stay there and focus on the action of your hips and pelvis to grind your pubic bone against her clit. You can also make use of the bed to create the back-and-forth grinding action you seek.

8. **The Ay Popi**—I came up with a few different names for this technique but settled on the Ay Popi in honor of my Latina fiancée, who happens to love when I do it to her . . . especially during anal sex! Basically, it calls for you to "pop" your penis in and out of the particular orifice you happen to be visiting at the moment. Varying the

depth of your insertion strokes will only add to her pleasure. This one's not for amateurs, however, as it takes a certain level of cock-eye coordination and aim to perform it properly or you could end up with a broken penis. I recommend slow, controlled strokes and using your hand to help guide it back into its glory hole. I am sure most of you don't know that if you come while doing this, it is no longer considered the Ay Popi. It would then be called the Popi Seed, of course!

9. **The Slaphappy**—This is a twist on the Ay Popi. It calls for you to pull completely out of her *pussy* and use your cock to slap or rub her pussy and clit before reinserting it again, thrusting some, and repeating the process. Notice I have emphasized the word "pussy" above. That's because it's probably not the best idea to do this during anal sex for reasons of health and hygiene.

10. **The Beat Box**—Throw on some music you both like and start pumping your hips to the rhythm of the beat. Or you could simply conjure up a favorite song in your head and start thrusting away. If your partner is good, she'll be able to name that tune in ten strokes or less.

11. **Missionary with a Twist**—This is a variation of the standard missionary position wherein the man places his legs on the outside of his partner's, while she spreads her legs only enough to allow his penis to enter her vagina. This will not only change up the angle of penetration and vary the stimulation for her, but it will also result in an added amount of dick friction for you.

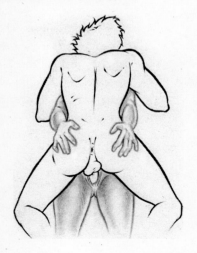

There you have the techniques I recommend you use during intercourse. As I have tried to get across to you, different women will respond differently to each technique. It's up to you to discover which works best for any particular partner. I encourage you to experiment with each technique and to be creative in your use of them. Adding your own touch to any of my suggestions in order to accommodate a specific partner is highly recommended! Also, using the techniques in combinations can elicit great responses. For example, mixing a dash of the Daily Grind with the Deep Six or a helping of the Shortstop with the Longfellow could be surefire recipes for satisfying her sexual appetite.

Now let's take a moment to probe deeper into specifically reaching and stimulating her G-spot with your penis. As you will see, this is more about positioning and angle of thrust than anything else.

Missionary—First a quick trick to improve the missionary experience. You and your partner may find it helpful if a pillow or two is placed beneath her ass. This will give her more freedom of hip movement and take any strain off her lower back. It also allows for easier and deeper penetra-

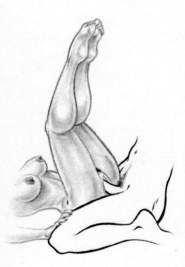

tion for you by elevating your partner's pussy or ass. Because the pillows are causing her pelvis to tip back, G-spot contact is more likely. Now, to access her G-spot while she is on her back, it is best to have her bring her legs back into her chest or over your shoulders. This will expose her spot more and make it easier to stimulate whether you're laying flat on top of her or approaching her on your knees with an upright torso. When you are on your knees you should try to lean back slightly so your penis is thrusting at an upward angle, which will apply pressure and stimulation to the upper wall of the orifice you happen to be visiting at the moment. Using the same technique during anal sex can produce similar results, as the membrane dividing her ass and pussy is very thin.

Reverse Cowgirl—In this position, the stimulation to the G-spot varies depending upon the actions of your partner. If she leans back, your penis will be applying pressure to her G-spot by rubbing over its outer surface as it travels along the upper wall of her love canal. If she leans slightly forward, a more direct poking or tapping type of stimulation will be achieved. Once on top of you, her actions will dictate which she prefers . . . which, of course, you will make a mental note of!

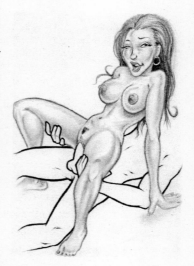

Doggie Style—While you can stimulate her G-spot in most variations of this position, up-and-over is the most effective variation. The higher you ride her, the better! This increases the downward pressure being applied and results in a more direct stimulation of her G-spot. Of course, the higher you ride her, the more your thighs will feel like a catcher's during an extra-innings baseball game. Nothing will make your thighs burn like ten minutes of up-and-over. The good news is that if you hit her spot just right she could ejaculate enough to douse those flames and make you forget all about the pain.

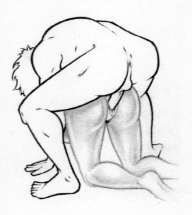

Pancake—This is another position that can be benefited by adding pillows. In this case, you would place them under her hips/lower abdomen as she lies facedown on top of them. Here you're looking for the same downward pressure as with doggie

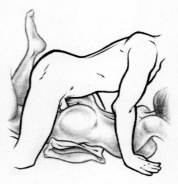

There are an estimated one hundred million acts of sexual intercourse each day.

style. Again, the higher you're able to ride her, the more directly you'll be able to stimulate her G-spot.

The last instruments that you need to get in tune with the rest of the orchestra are your fingers. Like a conductor's wand, your fingers have the ability to produce beautiful music—like the sounds of pure ecstasy as your partner delivers an orgasmic symphony in your ear. Women appreciate men who can multitask and innovate. So, whether you want to rub or slap her clit with your fingertips during intercourse or insert your fingers in her pussy or ass, here are some of the best positions for you to experiment with:

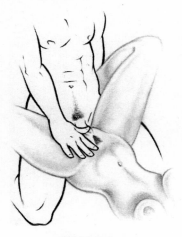

Missionary

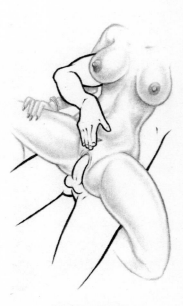

Reverse cowgirl

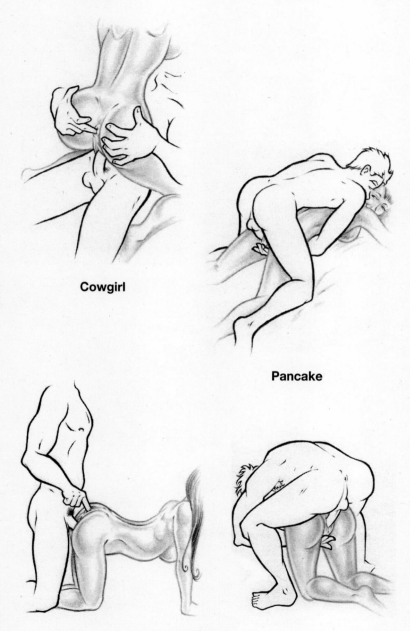

Cowgirl

Pancake

Doggie

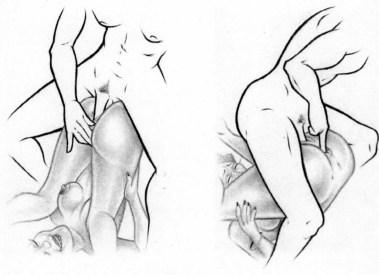

Pile driver

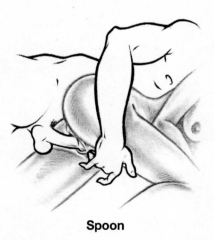

Spoon

Here are a few more positions that have drawn rave reviews from many of the women I have had the pleasure of spending sexy time with. As with a master magician, timing is everything. It's up to you to determine the right moment to pull a squatting rabbit out of your hat.

1. **Hiding Ostrich**—While requiring a touch of flexibility on your lover's part, this one offers maximum penetration. It provides you with direct access to her asshole and breasts plus reacharound access to her clit. Remember to hold on to her tight or you could knock her onto her head.

2. **Push Me Pull Me**—In this position, movement can be controlled by both you and your partner. As you pull her close to you, penetration becomes deeper. The intimacy factor is high because you are able to maintain eye contact and have direct access to her love button.

3. **Squatting Rabbit**—This is a great position for slow, romantic grinding. Once you are deeply inserted into her vagina or anus, your partner only needs to hold her position and slowly grind her hips into you. It makes for an excellent change of pace from the harder doggie position and will provide you with excellent access to kiss, fondle, or reach around her hip and masturbate her.

4. **Drunken Frog**—The trick to getting into this one is for you to lift your legs straight in the air while your partner, on her knees, pulls your cock forward and inserts it. Once inserted, you can then lower your legs and rest them around her thighs. This is another position dependent on the woman's ability to push back and grind herself on you.

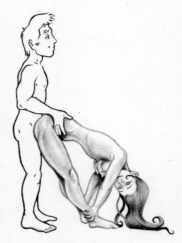

Hiding Ostrich

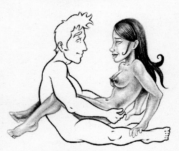

Push Me Pull Me

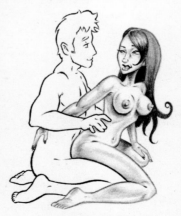

Squatting Rabbit

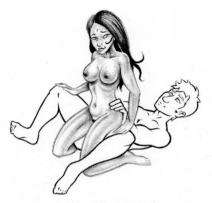

Drunken Frog

5. **Bouncing Frog**—This one is similar to the above but instead of your partner starting out on her knees, her feet are flat and she squats down on your dick. This gives her the ability to lean forward on her hands and bounce herself up and down your bean stalk.

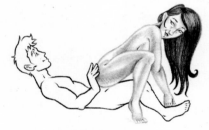

Bouncing Frog

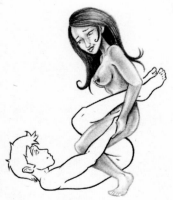

Tangled Crab

6. **Tangled Crab**—Here you lie on your back and raise your legs while your partner squats over your flagpole and inserts it as she faces you. The farther you get your legs back, the more freedom of movement she'll have.

7. **Rooster Tail**—This is an easy position to transition into from standard missionary and provides for maximum

penetration. It puts her in an excellent position for G-spot stimulation and makes for a nice change of pace. You can pound away or encourage her to grind herself against you by helping her lift and lower while she uses her arms for support and her ankles on your shoulders for leverage.

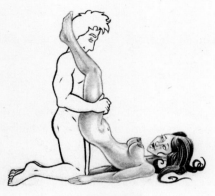

Rooster Tail

Adding some or all of the techniques we've discussed here to your repertoire will let your partner know she's not dealing with a novice. Combine them with all the other tips and tricks you should pick up from this book and you could be hearing the words "You're the best" sooner than you think!

Sexual Incompatibility

One of the most difficult aspects of writing this book is the need to generalize in order to speak to the "masses." I find myself using phrases like "most women" or "many of you men" as opposed to being able to speak to you as individuals and address each and every potential solution to

"I'd like to meet the man who invented sex and see what he's working on now."—Unknown

According to research, if you have sex one or two times per week, you are less likely to get sick.

"Love is a matter of chemistry but sex is a matter of physics."
—Unknown

each and every potential problem that can become an issue for a man. If I didn't generalize, this book would end up over a thousand pages long— and reading that many pages of anything written by someone like me would likely make your eyes bleed. The statement "Size doesn't matter to women" is clearly a generalization, as there are more than a few for whom size is of great importance, which brings me to the subject of sexual incompatibility. This is a very difficult issue for a couple to overcome and can cause frustration and a lowering of self-esteem in many cases. While I'm all about perseverance and the "where there's a will, there's a way" type of thinking, I also know there are times you have to simply accept things you don't like and move on. Trying to force compatibility is generally a losing proposition. Here are a few examples of what I'm talking about:

Physical Incompatibility

- A man with an extra-long penis and a woman with a super-shallow cervix.
- A man with an anal sex preference and a woman with irritable bowel syndrome (IBS) or Crohn's disease.

Mental Incompatibility

- A man who prefers rough sex and a woman who has experienced rape or sexual abuse in her past.

"Sex is as important as eating or drinking and we ought to allow the one appetite to be satisfied with as little restraint and false modesty as the other."—Marquis de Sade

Having sex three times per week for one year is equal to running seventy-five miles.

- A man who prefers to be submissive during sex and a woman who prefers to be submissive during sex.

Sadly, because many of us rush into sex without really getting to know our partners, we don't discover these roadblocks until after we've had sex or become emotionally invested in the relationship. Or some of us may see the red flags flying and choose to ignore them. If, for example, you are a five-foot-eight Caucasian guy with a four-inch cock and during your pursuit of a particular woman you find out that she has only previously dated extremely tall, well-hung African-American men—well, you're probably barking up the wrong vagina! Just like a woman with size-12 Fred Flintstone feet probably wouldn't have a lot of luck enticing a male with a dainty foot fetish.

CHAPTER 22

Anal Retention

You will encounter two types of women: those who are open to the idea of anal sex but inexperienced, and women who seem to be closed to the idea. The process of introducing either to anal sex is basically the same, except you will need to take a few extra steps with the latter. I'm going to lay it out step by step on the assumption that you are dealing with a "closed-minded" woman and let you decide the appropriate place to start:

STEP 1: GIVE HER A REASON

If you're expecting a woman to give you something that she hasn't given any other man, namely her asshole, you better be prepared to give her a good reason. I'm not talking about a four-karat rock, although that certainly couldn't hurt. I am talking about expressing yourself and letting her know how much you want to have anal sex with her. I am talking about paying particular attention to her ass, about showing her that you are just as interested in what turns her on and that you will make sure it's pleasurable for her, too.

STEP 2: PLANTING THE ANAL SEEDS

A woman could be closed to the idea of anal sex because she's had a bad experience with it in the past or because she's simply never been given a reason to associate anal sex with pleasure. One way to try to overcome this is by exposing your partner to other women who *enjoy* anal sex. This can be done by exposing her to a particular book or X-rated movie. Reading about other women having pleasurable anal experiences or actually watching other women have orgasms while having anal sex will help by providing her with a different, anal-positive perspective. If your partner enjoys reading, I highly recommend a book called *The Surrender* by Toni Bentley. It is the true story of a former ballerina whose life changes after she is introduced to anal sex. If your partner enjoys the occasional adult movie, I can proudly recommend any of my anal-themed movies, as they always feature girls who truly enjoy their work—getting fucked in the ass! I will caution you, though, that my movies leave absolutely nothing to the imagination! There is also a DVD called *Tristan Taormino's Expert Guide to Anal Sex* that I would highly recommend. Another way to "plant the seed" would be establishing new types of contact with her ass during sex. This could mean gently brushing your tongue across her butthole while you're going down on her or even sticking it all the way up her ass. This could mean using your fingertips to apply pressure to the outside of her anus during oral sex or intercourse. Or you could simply give her an anal massage as a part of foreplay. Again, using your fingertips, you would apply various amounts of pressure to her sphincter and taint.

STEP 3: ESTABLISH THE CONNECTION
It's important that you establish the connection between her ass and the concept of pleasure. I would recommend going about this in one of two ways, depending on your partner. If you are able to get her off by going down on her, this is probably the best way to proceed. You simply eat her pussy until she is on the verge of orgasm, at which point you gently insert a well-lubricated finger into her butt, working it in slowly, as you continue eating her pussy until she climaxes.

The other way you could approach it is while she masturbates. Take position between her legs as she buzzes her love button and plays with her pussy while you occasionally kiss her inner thighs. Ask her to tell you when she is about to come, and when she gives the word, slowly insert a well-lubricated finger into her butthole. You don't have to move it much;

Olive oil has been used as a sexual lubricant since 350 B.C.

just the fact that there is something stimulating her asshole during orgasm is more than enough to make the connection you're looking for.

STEP 4: PREPARATION A

This is the time, if you are able to get her to commit to letting you in her back door, that you will begin the "Anal Orientation" process.

First, you will need to make sure you have the following items:

One enema (you can get these at any drug- or grocery store)
One bottle of silicone-based lubricant (unless you're using latex
    condoms, in which case you need a water-based lubricant)
One small butt plug
One medium butt plug
One vibrator (a Pocket Rocket, for example)
One bottle of baby shampoo

Now, here is an example of a five-day anal orientation program (These five days should be spread out over a ten-to-twelve-day period.):

For days one through four you will instruct your partner to coat her index finger with the baby shampoo and use it to clean herself by inserting it in her ass and moving it in and out while showering before sex. However, she will need to do an enema before the big event on day five. One word of caution when it comes to enemas—you shouldn't assume that your partner knows how to use them. I can remember, back about six or seven years ago, a day I was scheduled to shoot a girl's first anal scene. Her name was Brandi, and she was a naturally large-breasted redhead with a genuine fire crotch. She was about twenty-two and had only been in the adult business a couple of weeks. Brandi's costar that day was a muscular black guy named Ronny, and, yes, he had quite the large cock. Brandi actually requested him, which at the time I found surprising considering the size of Ronny's schlong. I even said something to her, to which she replied, "Don't worry, I've been practicing with a big dildo for weeks."

Anyway, after makeup, Brandi was handed an enema by one of my

"Open her mind and her ass will follow."—Seymore Butts

production assistants and told to take care of her "girl stuff" in the bathroom because we were almost ready to start shooting. About fifteen minutes later, we went through some last-minute position discussions and we were rolling. Soon, Brandi was kissing her way down Ronny's body, unleashing his one-eyed monster as she traveled south. He was hard as a tire iron as Brandi sank to her knees and placed her hands behind her back while taking his cock in her mouth. With each movement of her head, she would try taking his dick in a little deeper. Finally, as she was trying to force the last few centimeters down her throat, she gagged and vomited so violently it was as if she was trying to exorcise the devil out of herself. After she stopped spasming, the conversation went like this:

Brandi: Holy shit, I'm so sorry! That's never happened before.
Me: Did you eat something before the scene?
Brandi: No way—you told me not to. I think it was the enema. It tasted like shit and I started feeling nauseous right when we started shooting.
Me: You drank the enema?
Brandi: Yeah, is that bad?

Looking back now, I find it funny, but the cleanup and resulting delays cost me time and money. The point is, make sure she's clear on how the whole enema thing works before you suggest she do one.

DAY ONE

After she has showered and cleaned herself as described, proceed with the sexual encounter as you would normally. The only thing you need to accomplish is to reaffirm the pleasure connection that you previously established. Again, you would do this by inserting a finger or small butt plug into her butthole as she is on the verge of orgasm as a result of oral sex or masturbation.

DAY TWO

Do everything that I mentioned in day one, except today you will also be introducing the small butt plug to her by inserting it into her ass before engaging in vaginal sex. Leave it in for the entire duration of the intercourse.

DAY THREE

Today you will do exactly the same things as day two, except you will substitute the medium-sized butt plug into the action.

DAY FOUR

Today you will repeat day three. (This doesn't mean you have to put her into the exact same positions when you're fucking her!)

DAY FIVE

This is the big day, which means you will both have to approach things a little differently. First, she should try to avoid eating for a period of five to six hours before showtime. This is not the day to take her to a chili cook-off. She should use the enema about four hours before the impending anal encounter. At this time, she should use the enema with the medicated solution. She should repeat the process again about an hour before blast-off, but this time filling the enema bottle with tap water. Have her top it all off with a pregame shower and final finger inspection—and she should be feeling more than confident that she's clean as a whistle! That's going to go a long way toward helping her be able to relax while you're busy stretching her sphincter to new proportions. By the way, unless you're prepared to go through a hell of a lot of bedsheets, this cleaning regimen or something similar that your partner finds effective should be done every time you have anal sex, not just the first few times. Now you're ready to repeat everything you did on day four. Of course, you will be adding a slight variation by removing the butt plug after intercourse and replacing it with your well-lubricated penis. Now is also the time you will introduce the vibrator into play by telling her to use it on her clit as you slowly enter her ass. Missionary or spoon is probably your best bet for "anal initiation" purposes. I know you would think doggie to be one of the better positions, but it actually enables the deepest penetration—and deepest isn't the best for anal newbies.

Depending on your partner's anal capacity, there is a possibility you may have to repeat your actions from day five a couple of times before you're really able to rock her tushy. It's also a good idea to maintain a semiregular anal schedule, at the least for a few weeks after the initiation. This will help build an anal tolerance, if you will, that will help ensure a lifetime of anal pleasure for you both.

There is another type of product I have found to be especially effective in helping to stretch a woman's anus in preparation for anal sex: the inflatable butt plug. This is a hollow butt plug that has a tube attached with a squeeze ball at the other end. You insert the uninflated plug into your partner's tushy and gradually inflate it as she gets comfortable with its increasing size. I've actually recommended this to many female adult performers—and it almost always received fantasstic reviews. One such girl was Sophie Dee. Now, Sophie can regularly be seen in my movies easily taking and genuinely enjoying the largest of cocks up her beautiful British bum. She wasn't always so anally receptive, though—she certainly wasn't the British lass who loves it in the ass that she is now.

Sophie actually did her first anal scene in one of my movies, and it was asstounding—but in all honesty, it was her second attempt at the feat. We had to cancel the first attempt because something went terribly wrong on set that day. It started out great—everyone arrived on time, Sophie was extremely excited, and our male talent was hard as he walked in the door, knowing that he was going to be the first to stretch out Sophie's virgin arse (getting the call to do a girl's first anything is considered a badge of honor among male porn stars). Anyhow, after makeup, Sophie announced that she was going to do her "girlie stuff" and then proudly pulled an inflatable butt plug out of her bag, mentioned how she'd been practicing, and reiterated how excited she was as she tittered out of the room. Fast-forward about thirty-five minutes when I heard Sophie let out a blood-curdling scream. I ran into the room to find Sophie on the bed with the butt plug in one hand while her other hand was covering her asshole.

Me: What happened?

Sophie: I'm too embarrassed to tell you.

Me: Embarrassed? Are you OK? What did you do?

Sophie: When I used this thing at home, I was never able to get past four squeezes, and today I got to seven squeezes. I got so excited; I never thought that I could get to seven squeezes. I was dying to see how big it got, so I just pulled it out without deflating it first and I think I ripped my poor little butthole!

You're damn right she ripped it! After seven squeezes, it must have been like yanking a grapefruit out of her rectum. Canceling that shoot was definitely a pain in my ass but it was certainly nothing compared to what Sophie was going through! After the initial disappointment faded, both Sophie and I couldn't help but find some humor in the situation and shared a good laugh. Thankfully, she recovered within a few weeks and was determined to give it another shot—this time hitting it in the dead center of the ~~brown eye~~, er, I mean bull's-eye!

Some women might worry that frequent anal sex will stretch their buttholes out to the point of needing to wear diapers. The fact is, assholes have a great amount of elasticity. Unless a woman is into inserting extremely large objects like baseball bats or champagne bottles into her anus on a regular basis, this should not be a concern.

I have met a lot of women in my day who have had a lot of anal sex. While I have yet to meet a woman who needed to wear diapers as a result of engaging in anal sex, I have known some to have to deal with an occasional uprising of hemorrhoids. They are caused by excessive pressure in the rectum, which compels the blood vessels to expand and bulge the walls of veins around or inside the anus. Think of them like varicose veins of the rectum. There are two types of hemorrhoids, external and internal, which are classified by degrees. A first-degree hemorrhoid would be the least serious and most common—easily treated with over-the-counter medications like Preparation H. A fourth-degree hemorrhoid, also called a "prolapsed rectum," is the most serious, resulting in the bulging veins and surrounding tissue protruding from her anus. In other words, it looks like her asshole is turning inside out. This condition is usually the result of stretching the sphincter beyond normal, penis-sized proportions—if it's a result of anal sex, that is. You see, there are many other common causes of hemorrhoids, including:

Constant sitting
Excessive pushing during bowel movements due to constipation
Diarrhea
Severe coughing
Pregnancy/childbirth
Heavy lifting
Sitting on the toilet for long periods of time
Heredity
Aging

I wish I knew as much about hemorrhoids in 2003 as I do today. I'm thinking specifically of an October afternoon when I was shooting content for both my Web site and my television show, *Family Business,* simultaneously. It also happened to be a day when I had scheduled shooting two scenes, which is unusual for me. The set was more chaotic than it normally is. I had just finished shooting the first scene as I was approached by Crystal, the girl scheduled to perform in the second scene, which was supposed to be a boy/girl vaginal encounter with a heavy emphasis on oral sex and ass licking. This also happened to be the second scene of Crystal's adult film career. The attractive, blue-eyed blonde with large fake tits and a fitness model's body had recently left the strip clubs of the Midwest to pursue sexual stardom. She actually arrived on set early this day and had the opportunity to watch seasoned tushy girl Flower Tucci spray like a fire hose and call out to God while devouring a very large penis with her hungry asshole. I couldn't help but notice Crystal's hand conspicuously between her thighs as she sat off-camera and watched us film. Anyway, after Flower was properly pollinated, Crystal approached me and we had a conversation that went like this:

Crystal: Wow, that was so hot! I had no idea girls could get off like that from anal sex.
Me: Yeah, that did work out well.
Crystal: I kinda want to try it.

Me: Great, you can do it in my next movie.

Crystal: No, I mean I want to try it today. I was planning on start-ing to do it soon anyway.

Me: But you haven't prepped properly.

Crystal: My ex stuck his finger in there tons of times and I've even stuck my vibrator in there once.

Me: No, that's not really what I meant. There are certain things you should and shouldn't do before an anal scene. Most im-portantly, you really can't eat for hours before the scene.

Crystal: That's perfect, because I was so nervous about shooting for you that I haven't been able to eat since yesterday afternoon.

Me: Really?

Crystal: Really!

Me: I'll tell you what—give me five minutes to discuss it with Chris [her costar]. Meanwhile, you go take care of your girl stuff and do an enema with tap water. You do know how to do an enema?

Crystal: Of course! Great! Which bathroom can I use?

I pointed her in the right direction and went to find Chris. Sure, there are male performers in the industry who don't like anal sex and prefer to avoid it, but I knew Chris wasn't one of them—it was more of a courtesy gesture than anything. As I expected, Chris was more than agreeable and actually might have started to drool, if I remember correctly. I couldn't blame him, as the thought of Crystal's smooth, round, firm, perfectly shaped buttocks swallowing their penis would make many men drool. However, there had to be more factored into my decision than simply the stud's consent. I have shot many "anal debuts" during my career and have found them to be a very black and white, hit-or-miss type of proposition. It's either a sphinctacular success—which entails the actress actually en-joying the experience and the movie itself enjoying strong sales, because the porn consumer has shown a propensity for gravitating toward "mile-stone firsts," e.g., a girl's first scene, first interracial scene, first anal scene, etc.—or it's a major disaster, which could entail shouts of excruciating pain, tears, a bleeding butthole, or anal leakage. Any of these could result

"Don't worry, it only seems kinky the first time."—Unknown

in having to kill the scene and wasting the time and energy of all involved. I also needed to consider the fact that delaying Crystal's anal initiation for another day meant risking that that day might never come. After all, the average adult actress is only able to last about three months in the industry. There are a number of potential reasons for these shortened careers:

- A bad experience on set, e.g., the actress feels taken advantage of or the actress is physically injured in some way.
- Pressure to leave the industry from family and/or friends.
- Pressure to leave the industry from a new boyfriend.
- Child-custody issues force the actress to leave the industry.
- The actress comes to a quick realization that the industry is simply not for her.

No matter what the reason, the risk was real, as I had seen it happen many, many times. When I was a young man training to sell women's shoes, I was taught, "The be-back bus almost never comes back." In this particular situation, considering all of the above, Crystal's enthusiasm and especially the perfectly round symmetry of her world-class tushy each played a role in my decision to give Crystal the green light. I handed her a butt plug as I gave her the news and instructed her to insert it after she was done cleaning herself. Meanwhile, I had to tweak my shooting notes to incorporate the changes. Thirty-five minutes later, all principles were on set—prepped and blocked, waiting for my call. *"Action,"* I yelled as Chris positioned himself behind Crystal, kissing her neck and rubbing her breasts and pussy. I moved my camera in front of Crystal and concentrated on her facial reactions. Chris had taken her top off and dropped to his knees while he removed her skirt and panties. He kissed her buns a few times before spreading her cheeks and burying his face in her ass. The next thing I knew, Chris's head was peeking around Crystal's right hip with a look of horror. He was moving his mouth strangely. It took me a second to figure out he was trying to get me to read his lips—"Looook aat herr azzhole." Look at her asshole? I couldn't understand what the problem could be but I yelled, *"Cut!"* and asked Chris what the problem was. The *Family Business* cameras continued to roll during the following exchange:

> **Me:** What seems to be the problem?
> **Chris:** I think you should take a look at this.
> **Crystal:** What's wrong?
> **Me:** I'm sure it's nothing. Do me a favor, get on your hands and knees and spread your cheeks so I can get a look.

Crystal complied and I moved in for a closer examination. It's hard to describe what I saw. I had never seen anything like it before and have only seen it since in pictures on the Internet. It was a large, swollen, purplish, knobby mass protruding from her anus. It was quite ferocious-looking! Looking back, I should have, like the many before me who have discovered new species of life, taken the opportunity to name the monstrosity that was perched before me. If I did, I might have borrowed the nickname of the vaunted Minnesota Vikings defense of the 1970s, led by greats like Carl Eller and Alan Page, and dubbed it "the Purple People-Eater." Or I might have drawn from Hollywood and named it "Elephant Anus." All joking aside, although I didn't know it at the time, I was staring at a hemorrhoid of the fourth degree. Not having seen anything like it before, I really had no idea what to do. Of course, I didn't let Crystal know any of this. I acted completely calm and asked her a few questions:

> **Me:** You're sure you've never had anal sex before?
> **Crystal:** Of course I'm sure!
> **Me:** And you haven't had any pain down here lately?
> **Crystal:** No.
> **Me:** [touching the monster]Does this hurt?
> **Crystal:** No.

As I touched it more, I noticed I could actually push or tuck the purple monster back into her ass; however, a few seconds later it would inevitably pop out and rear its ugly head. Then I lubed up my index finger and

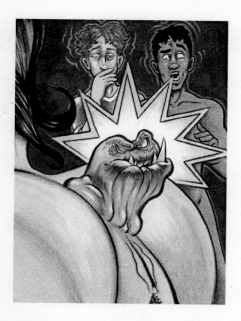

inserted it. I could see that the act of inserting my finger pushed the monster back into its hole. Unfortunately, the act of withdrawing my finger pulled it right back out again. I concluded that it would be best to kill the anal portion of the scene. I tried to minimize the situation for Crystal by telling her that she seemed to have a slight irritation around her asshole and she should have it checked out by her doctor. Her ass was so round and fleshy, I knew shooting around the purple mystery wouldn't be a problem for me—and it wasn't. The scene turned out great. Aside from Chris starting out a tad slow—he later explained it took him a few minutes to erase the vision of purple fury that had been temporarily burned into his brain—I would say it went perfectly. Sadly, I've never been able to muster the courage to invite Crystal back to shoot her anal scene. I've gotta believe she got a handle on her purple problem, because she's become known as a back-door queen of sorts and has performed in literally hundreds of anal scenes since.

Warning Warning Warning Warning Warning Warning Warning

When it comes to anal play and exploration, there is one thing you must always keep in mind: When using fingers, a toy, or your cock, you can go from her vagina to her ass but never, ever go from her ass to her vagina. Doing this can put your partner at risk of developing a serious bacterial infection called E. coli. The symptoms of this could include bloody diarrhea, cramps, nausea, fever, or vomiting. People who are infected with E. coli are highly contagious and need to be treated by a medical professional immediately!

In Case of Emergency

Unlike vaginal sex, where saliva can do in a pinch, only the most anally experienced woman can even think about butt sex without the help of a commercial lubricant. I'm sure you've heard the old Boy Scout motto "Always be prepared," but I bet you didn't know it was originally coined by scoutmasters to remind themselves to bring lube on the scouting jamborees. Anyway, if you ever happen to find yourself unprepared for an anal encounter, here are a few items that are likely to be found around anyone's home or hotel or can be purchased at a variety of retail outlets:

1. Olive oil—Extra-virgin, of course!
2. Crisco—A favorite of many gay men.
3. Butter—Infamously used by Marlon Brando to butt-fuck Maria Schneider in *Last Tango in Paris.*
4. Hair conditioner—Sometimes you have to think outside the box!
5. Albolene—This is sold at major drugstores as a makeup remover for women. It also makes for a great anal lubricant.

CHAPTER 23

Spanking Good Times

There are certain things that stand out in my mind—things I've heard, things I've seen, things I've done, etc.—and some of them I completely understand my retention of; as for others, I don't have a fucking clue as to why they would stand out to me above others.

For instance, I can look back to a two-minute slice of a particular day during my freshman year of high school and remember it vividly—because of an eight-word sentence I heard uttered that particular day. Class had just let out and I was moving along to my next class, part of the herd at Santa Monica High, when I found myself directly behind the two hottest girls in school. Terri and Dana were both seniors and complete physical opposites. Terri was Latina, with long dark hair, tan skin, and bright green eyes. Her C-cup tits and perky butt made her the total package in my opinion. I had a huge crush on her, but at the time, I would have never had the balls to approach her. She always seemed to have a boyfriend anyway. Dana was the prototypical California blonde and she could really surf too! They were in midconversation as I turned my ears to eavesdropping mode. This is what I heard:

Dana: You actually liked that?
Terri: Oh my god—it hurt so fuckin' good!
Dana: I knew you were a perv!
Terri: Oh, like you have any room to talk—like, gag me!

They both laughed and headed off in separate directions. I went on to class but couldn't get those eight words out of my head. They're still in my

"It is always by way of pain one arrives at pleasure."
—Marquis de Sade

head! I remember being so curious as to what Terri was talking about—what "hurt so fuckin' good"? Of course, I hoped she was talking about anal sex!

Fast-forward six years later. I was with some friends in a Santa Monica bar and who did I see but Terri and Dana—both looking great, I might add! Surprisingly, they recognized me—probably because I lived two blocks away from Dana during our high school years. I bought them some drinks and we did a little reminiscing before hitting the dance floor. Don't ask me how, because it certainly wasn't the result of any well-planned "move," but soon all three of us were making out on the dance floor. It's still, to this day, one of the single hottest moments in my life—probably because of the pedestal I had put them on in high school. There I was with two of the finest, most unattainable girls from high school taking turns shoving their tongues down my throat. My boys couldn't believe what they were seeing and the incident increased my street cred exponentially. Soon we would hear "Last call," at which time Dana left, saying she had to be at work early. Terri invited me back to her place, where I would later learn that Dana actually had to get home to her fiancé. Terri gave me a quickie tour of her apartment that culminated with us in her bedroom. After a little tonsil hockey, she grabbed something out of her dresser and excused herself to go to the bathroom. I bravely approached the bathroom door and initiated the following conversation:

Me: [*knock knock*] Hey, I got a question for you. It's been killing me since high school.
Terri: Yes?
Me: What "hurt so good"?
Terri: What?
Me: Do you remember a conversation you had in school with Dana where you said, "Oh my god—it hurt so fuckin' good!"?
[*Pause*]
Terri: Yeah, kinda, but how do you know about it?

Me: I was walking right behind you when you said it but I didn't hear the first part of the conversation and I've been dying to know ever since I heard you say it.

Terri: Wow, you have a good memory. Sooo [voice change], you want to know what I was talking about. What do you think I was talking about?

Me: To be honest, I hope you tell me you were taking it in the tushy.

Terri: Why? You like anal sex?

Me: Well, yeah, that and it kinda fit the dialogue.

Terri: I hate to disappoint you but it was actually the first time a guy spanked me during sex—and the first time I realized that I liked it!

Over that summer, Terri and I had numerous very intimate encounters during which I was able to learn how to spank a woman properly thanks to Terri's patience and guidance. Terri was a spanking fetishist—a true spankophile!

A spanking fetish is a sexual deviation (while this is the technical definition, enthusiasts would argue it's an art) where a person is sexually aroused by spankings—either on the receiving or giving end, or both. There are many theories as to why a person would develop a spanking fetish, with most of them tracing the deviation to experiences we have as children. Sigmund Freud believed that some children may deal with a painful or traumatic experience by "eroticizing" it. Others believe the physical pain induced by spanking causes an endorphin rush, like certain drugs, which some people may experience as a pleasurable sensation. If a child is spanked repeatedly, resulting in frequent, intense endorphin rushes, that child may become "addicted" to spankings. There are even those who believe the act of presenting the buttocks for a spanking resembles the pose that a female ape assumes during mating. Personally, I'm a believer that there is more than just a casual relationship between spanking and being physical with a child, and the sexual deviations that child may develop as a grown-up. That is one of the reasons I have never spanked my son.

There are many women who enjoy being spanked before, during, and after sex. We could probably spend a couple of chapters together trying to figure out exactly why, but in the end (every pun intended), does it really matter why they like it? Hell no! The only thing that really matters is that you have the ability to deliver a proper spanking when the moment calls for it. Here are some pointers on spanking that I've picked up over the years.

> Most people feel comfortable spanking with their dominant, more coordinated hand. Remember, some of the elements of giving a proper spanking include touch and aim.
>
> No matter which hand you decide to go with, make sure you warm it up real well before you lay it on her tushy.
>
> Whether you're spanking her sitting or standing, make sure you have ample room to raise your arm and maneuver freely.
>
> Place your fingers together tightly and slightly cup your hand before spanking her. This will ensure a mild but very pleasurable sting along with a nice clean smacking sound.
>
> Always aim for the fleshiest part of her ass. You want to avoid hitting her lower back or upper thighs. You should also avoid spanking both cheeks at the same time. You can alternate which cheek you spank, but don't hit them both simultaneously.
>
> Most accomplished spankers use no more than a one-to-two-foot backswing. That would be the farthest distance their hand would be from its target at any time.
>
> Responsible spankophiles will always use a "safe word." This is a word that participants in a spanking session agree to use to signify that the spanking is too hard and should be stopped.

Don't forget that women are as into the mental stimulation of the act as the physical sensations they feel. Most women will say they get as much out of the firm tone and direction they experience during the spanking as the spanking itself. In other words, don't let her forget who's in charge during these times. Asking her things like "Was that too hard?" is not going to cut the mustard. Part of being in control is observing her reactions and adjusting your actions according to your partner's individual threshold.

In addition to the bare hand, paddles, canes, riding crops, and even hairbrushes are widely used spanking implements. Avoid using paddles with holes, as they can inflict damage, such as blisters.

Positions that are most effective for spanking a woman properly include:

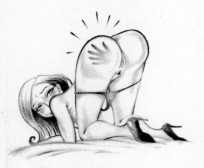

On hands and knees

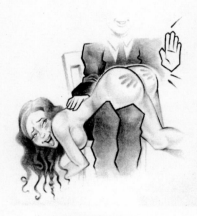

Across the lap

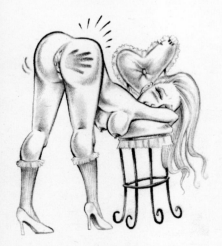

Bent over a chair or bench

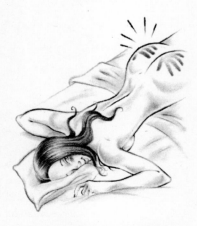

Lying facedown on the bed

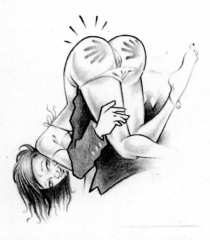

On the shoulder of the spanker

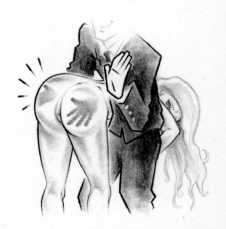

Bent under the arm of the spanker

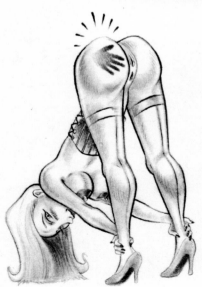

Standing and touching toes

Remember this stuff just in case you run into a girl like Terri! While this chapter is dedicated to a specific fetish, I want to take a moment to discuss fetishes in general.

What's a Fetish?

Sex professionals have different theories as to why we develop our fetishes. Many hours have been spent by many brilliant people to find the roots of our fetishes. I have only one question to ask you on the subject—do you really care? How much time do you spend wondering why you like chocolate ice cream but don't like strawberry ice cream? Why you like spicy food while others don't? How about why you prefer the color red to the color blue? I mean, do you really give a flying fuck? In my opinion, the word "fetish" is just a fancy way of describing a personal taste or preference. The only people who need to know the reason for their fetish are those whose preference or taste for something becomes an uncontrollable compulsion. This applies to food, drugs, gambling, exercise, masturbation, sex, and many other things. Other than that, if you have a preference for tall redheads with three nipples, fat feet, and thunder thighs while I have a preference for petite brunettes with big tits and round asses, so what? You should never let yourself feel guilty for having a particular taste, preference, fetish—whatever you want to call it. It's one of the things that makes you, you. Now you just have to make sure that you spend your time with women who appreciate you and the rest should come easy!

"To know what you prefer, instead of humbly saying 'amen' to what the world tells you you ought to prefer, is to keep your soul alive."—Robert Louis Stevenson

Approximately one out of every two hundred women is born with a third nipple.

CHAPTER 24

Throw Her a Curveball

Like a power pitcher who extends his career by adding an assortment of off-speed pitches to his repertoire, keeping your sexual activities fresh and exciting is key to maintaining a long-term, happy, healthy relationship. Below is a list of some things you can do to spark your sex life. The list is really recommended for those of you who know your partner well and have had sex with her on multiple occasions, as pulling any of these stunts during a first-time encounter would probably be pushing it—at least with a sober partner!

Depending on the type of sexual relationship you have with your partner, things such as eating her pussy, sticking a finger in her ass, or bringing home an adult movie could be considered "throwing her a curveball." In comparison, this list is probably best for those of you whose relationships are more advanced—at least sexually.

Hot Times—Buy a bottle of that lubrication that gets warm after you apply it. Without telling her, switch it up with your regular lube one night and watch for her reaction.

Pussy Sneak Attack—The idea here is to surprise her by playing with her pussy when she is not expecting it. For example, wait until you notice she is wearing a skirt when you are in your car driving somewhere and reach your hand over to her thigh and start gently caressing it as you make your way up to her pussy. And don't forget to keep your eyes on the road! Another variation of this concept would be to wait until you notice her

"The backseat produced the sexual revolution."—Jerry Rubin

wearing a skirt to the movies. Make sure you get yourself a drink with extra ice. Sometime after the lights go down, sneak an ice cube from your cup into your hand and start by rubbing it along her inner thigh. By the time you get to her love button, she'll be begging you to stick a few ice cubes inside of her.

Take Her for a Spin—Take her by surprise while she's doing the laundry. Put her up on the washing machine and show her what the spin cycle was really meant for!

Quickie Time—Drive her to a deserted, scenic spot and invite her into the backseat with you to share her favorite alcoholic beverage, which you just so happen to have chilling in a cooler in the trunk. Of course, parking lots, public restrooms, dressing rooms, and stairwells will do in a quickie pinch as well!

Shave Her Pussy and Ass—Many women enjoy the experience of being shaved by a man. They find it sensual and dangerous at the same time. Now, if you are going to shave her, make sure you are using a good-quality safety razor with a new, sharp blade. You will also need shaving cream or soap, a small amount of toilet tissue (I hope you only need a small amount), and some baby oil. Before you start, you'll need to fill a sink with hot water and place the shaving cream can and baby oil bottle in the water. The first thing to do is trim her bush. Begin by placing a towel under her and then use a comb to run gently through her pubic hair to remove tangles. Now, using a pair of small scissors with rounded ends (or with adhesive tape covering sharp ends), trim her bush as short as you can with the scissors. Next, lay a warm washcloth over her entire pussy and leave it there while you retrieve the shaving cream can from the sink. Remove the washcloth and apply the shaving cream liberally over her pubic mound and labia. Try to avoid putting the shaving cream over her clit and inner labia, so you can clearly see them to avoid them with the razor. Now, dip the razor in warm water, dab it dry on a towel, and start with light, even strokes while holding her skin taut with your other hand. When you approach those sensitive areas I mentioned, try using your own finger to cover and protect them from being nicked. If you do happen to spot a cut, put a dry piece of toilet paper on it, just as you would if you had cut yourself shaving your face, and continue on. Always try to shave in the same direction as the hair growth and avoid passing the razor over the same area repeatedly, as both will help her to avoid skin irritation. Once you are done, take the warm baby oil and massage it in all around the area you just shaved. If you want to shave her tushy, just flip her over onto all fours and repeat the process. Look, if this is something that is appealing to you and you're waiting for your partner to one day come out of the blue and ask, "Honey, do you want to shave my pussy?" I'm here to tell you the odds of that happening are slim to none. Nor will you be shaving your partner's pussy any time soon unless you just man up and tell her that's what you want to do!

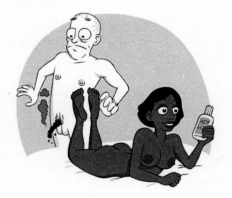

"Wow, this warming lube
really works!"

Better Sex—Invite her to watch a sporting event with you and propose a wager of a sexual nature. For example, you ask her to choose the team she thinks will win the game. You'll agree to take the other team. Whoever's team loses will need to perform thirty minutes of unreciprocated oral sex on the winner. This is something you sports nuts should be able to get creative with. And who knows—if you lose enough you might even turn her into a sports fan!

Make Your Own Dirty Movie—This can be a fun and intimate experience for both of you during the actual filming and also when you watch it together. As I mentioned in the introduction, I have made a movie for amateur filmmakers called *Do-It-Yourself Porn,* which gives a variety of instructions on how to give your amateur productions a professional touch. Of course, if you're a celebrity or a politician, I would avoid making any appearances in such a production . . . unless you want to sell me the rights!

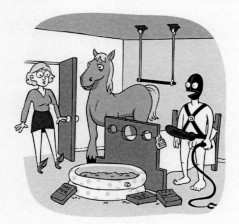

"Well, you said you wanted to
'spice things up a little,' right?"

Fruity Patooty—For this game, you will need to blindfold your partner. Now you'll be inserting various fruits or vegetables (for the more adventurous) into your partner's tunnel of love and challenging her to identify them. Strawberries, grapes, cherries, bananas, cucumbers, zucchinis, and carrots are especially conducive to this game.

Deep Freeze—Like the Fruity Patooty, this involves fun with foreign objects. This time I'm referring to phallic-shaped popsicles—a personal favorite of some of my ex-lovers. You can also find tubular ice trays, at Wal-Mart for instance, that also work well for this type of sex play.

Moving Violation—Hire a limo for the night and instruct the driver to travel along the most scenic routes in your area. Then it's time to pop the champagne, throw off your clothes, and enjoy both rides!

Good Vibes—Let her know you're taking her out on the town. Make sure you give her plenty of advance warning; women need notice, if you haven't noticed. Wait until the last possible minute before your departure to spring a pair of vibrating panties on her. Ask her to put them on while you explain that you will be holding the remote control all evening. Just the suspense of not knowing when she's gonna get "buzzed" is going to keep her turned on all night. If you take her to dinner, make sure you don't miss the opportunity to buzz her while she's placing her order with your waiter! Just make sure she doesn't get too carried away with her new toy, like the thirty-three-year-old woman who decided to wear a pair to the grocery store. Apparently, she became so overwhelmed with the phallic symbolism in the produce department, she fainted—hitting her head and knocking herself unconscious. When the paramedics arrived, they found her panties were still vibrating!

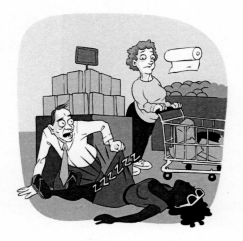

"It's OK—I'm a doctor!'"

Sex on the Beach—Most women have romantic notions of beaches and oceans. Just make sure you arrive prepared. Here is a checklist to keep in mind:

Blankets: You should have at least two blankets with you, one to lay underneath you and one to place over you in case it gets cold. This is imperative if you want to avoid getting a lot more gritty than nitty when you're getting down to the nitty-gritty.

Drink/Snacks: It's natural to get thirsty during sex and the munchies afterward. Hey, if you're gonna do it, do it right!

Bottle Opener/Corkscrew: There's nothing like pulling out a couple of beers or a nice bottle of wine and having no way to open them.

Flashlight: I'm assuming that most of you would attempt something like this at night. Depending on the type of terrain you have to negotiate to get to your oceanfront destination, a flashlight can come in very handy in guiding your partner safely back home.

Self-Defense Weapon: Whether it's pepper spray, a stun gun, or whatever, it's always good to carry a legal self-defense weapon with you. Anytime you engage in intimate behavior in public you are putting yourself and your partner at risk of not only arrest but attack.

Choose your destination carefully: The simple fact is that some beaches are closed at night. Make sure the beach you choose is accessible to the public at night or you risk an experience similar to one I had back in 1979.

It was a cool summer night during the fifteenth year of my existence. I was very excited getting ready for the evening as I was about to spend some alone time with a girl I had been interested in for a while. Her name was Britt and she was a natural blonde of Swedish descent. She stood about five foot four, with small pert breasts and the type of round, firm ass that always whooshes blood to my nether regions. After showering, I threw on my favorite jeans and T-shirt but found myself waffling between a hoodie and leather jacket. Usually, I wouldn't have given it a second thought, but tonight was different. It was special—at least I hoped it would be. Then it struck me: My dad's green sweater—actually, his very favorite golfing sweater—would be perfect. I swear if he was home, I would have asked his permission . . . but he wasn't, so I didn't. I was out of the house by six forty-five P.M., hopped on my bike, and started peddling. I gotta say I was looking good in that green sweater—there was no way Britt would be able to resist me. I rode down Montana Avenue and made a quick stop at a buddy's house to "borrow" a bottle of wine; my parents weren't drinkers, and neither was I for that matter, but I knew Britt liked her alcoholic beverages. I arrived at her house around seven thirty P.M. and found her waiting for me, in painted-on jeans, on her front steps. She jumped up on my handlebars and we were off. Britt lived only about seven blocks from the beach so it wasn't long before we were locking up my bike and strolling across the beach looking for a place to get cozy. It wasn't until we were actually under lifeguard station number 8 that I suddenly realized I was grossly unprepared for the evening I had imagined. My two biggest mistakes were forgetting both a blanket and a corkscrew. I solved the blanket problem quickly by taking off my—or should I say my dad's—sweater and laying it down on the sand for Britt to sit on. Solving the corkscrew problem proved to be a lot more difficult but I eventually broke the top half of the cork off and pushed the remaining end in the bottle. Of course, I didn't bring any glasses either, so we were forced to swig straight from the bottle. That is, Britt was forced to swig from the bottle and I was forced to act like I was drinking. Like I said, I wasn't a drinker. However, I felt it would be rude to allow her to feel as if she was drinking alone, so every time she passed me the bottle, I would put it to my tight lips, tip it, and dry-swallow a few times. She must have liked the wine because "we" finished the bottle off in less than ten minutes—and then things began to heat up under lifeguard station number 8! It started with some serious macking and within minutes we were both half-naked and Britt was pulling me on top of her, telling me, "I want to feel you inside me." She didn't have to ask twice and I slid my penis inside her very, very wet pussy. I remember thinking how good it felt and that I wanted it to last. That's why I moved in and out of her so slowly at first and tried concentrating on how good her lips felt as I kissed them or the sound of the waves crashing or the strong sea air smell—anything but how good that warm, wet pussy felt. And there we were starting to get into a slow, intense rhythm. Just as her breathing started to get heavy and her moans were getting louder, I was startled by a bright light shining in my eyes and the sound of a loud voice over an intercom:

"This is the police. This beach is restricted at night. You are trespassing and will need to leave now!"

Like a deer in headlights, I was frozen, until Britt hit me on the

"It is often said that men are ruled by their imaginations; but it would be truer to say they are governed by the weakness of their imaginations."—Walter Bagehot

shoulder and asked, "What are we going to do?" My mind raced for a moment until I blurted, "Is it cool if we take a few minutes to finish?" Hey, I didn't know if I was ever gonna get this opportunity again—and I really wanted to come—but sadly the cops weren't sympathetic to my cause and responded with a resounding, "No, you must leave the area now or you will be arrested." So we hurriedly got dressed and headed for my bike. By this time it was past nine, Britt and I were both a little rattled, and we decided to call it a night. I dropped Britt off and decided to head over to the Duck Blind liquor store to pick up a snack and a drink. I wasn't twenty yards away from Britt's when I noticed that same strong odor from the beach as if it were following me. I parked my bike outside the Duck Blind, untied the sweater from around my waist, and put it on as I entered the store. I immediately noticed two things—a friend of mine was playing video games and the place smelled something like I'd imagine the balls of an old fisherman with chronic jock itch might. So I approached my friend and after the obligatory "What's up, dude?" asked, "What the fuck's that smell?" And he looked at me kinda funny. "Dude, you don't smell that?" I asked again. He took a deep sniff of the air and I could tell by the look on his face he now knew what I was talking about. He sniffed again and then some more, letting his nose lead him like a bloodhound until it stopped him less than an inch away from my chest, or should I say my dad's very favorite green Lacoste golf sweater. It was just at this moment that I looked down and noticed a large dark area covering the chest of the sweater, which was also the moment that my buddy snapped his head away from me and said, "It's you, man! You smell like a sperm whale fart." "How could it be me?" I thought. "Impossible!" Then I put my hand to the dark area on my chest and felt it was damp. Then I brought the chest of the sweater to my nose and I nearly passed out. My friend was brave enough to give it another sniff and said, "That seriously smells like some gnarly pussy stank!" Then it struck me: Holy mackerel, it was Britt—we had sex on my dad's green sweater. I told you her pussy was wet, I just had no idea it was infected (now I know she had a very bad bacterial infection). I started to panic, wondering what I was going to do. I knew my dad would be super-pissed if he found out what happened. I decided to ride over to my buddy's where I had picked up the wine and ask to borrow his washer and dryer. I figured I could clean the sweater and have it back in my dad's closet before he knew it was ever gone. Needless to say, I figured wrong. Who knew sweaters aren't meant to be put in dryers? I can safely say it's the only time in my life that I wished my father was a midget. I ended up throwing it in a trash can and playing completely ignorant when the case of the missing green sweater became the main topic of discussion at home. If only I'd brought a blanket—my dad would still be wearing his very favorite green Lacoste sweater on the links today.

AUTHOR'S NOTE

To my father, who will undoubtedly get wind of this:

Hey, Dad,

Sorry about the sweater! I should have said something but I couldn't find the words. At least you can now consider the case closed!

Blow Her Pussy Up—This is where you take a small firecracker, also known as a "ladyfinger," and insert it inside her . . . just kidding! Seriously, though, there is a type of sex play referred to as female pumping. It is done by applying a vacuum suction device to pussies, clits, tits, and even assholes. This will cause the targeted body part to swell and engorge with blood, making it extra-sensitive to stimulation. Some women take pumping further and use it to actually increase the length of their nipples, for instance, by constantly pumping them over a period of time. You can learn more about safe female pumping techniques and where to buy the equipment needed to get started at Femalepumping.net.

Do-It-Yourself Dildo—Maybe you're about to leave on a long business trip or maybe your partner is going away for a while . . . nothing says "I love you and I'm going to miss you" like giving her a functional replica of your cock! There are products available now that enable you to make yourself into a dildo. I can hear a few of you saying, "I get called a dildo all the time, what's the big deal?" Seriously, if you Google "make your own dildo" you will find several products that will be the type of gift that keeps on giving and will ensure that you will be on her mind, or at least in her pussy, while you two are separated. In case you're wondering about the possibility of taking her pussy on the road with you, just Google "clone a vagina." With each of you equipped with the other's replica genitals, you'll literally be able to fuck each other from opposite ends of the earth.

The Fist Amendment—This is definitely not for everyone. Fisting is the act of inserting one's entire hand, usually balled up in a fist, into the sexual orifice of your partner. Ideally, the woman is stimulated by the idea of being penetrated by something so large as well as the physical sensation of being slowly and methodically stretched beyond her imagination. It also has proven to be a very satisfying, highly erotic experience for the man doing the fisting.

Personally, I enjoy the whole process of working my partner's vagina until it is finally able to accommodate my whole hand. Though the best part to me is when I'm able to start moving my fist in and out while watching my partner writhe in ecstasy. It's a very powerful, dominant kind of feeling. It's also another great way to simulate that "big dick" experience I spoke of in chapter 5. For women who have extremely narrow or tight vaginal canals and for guys with oven mitts for hands, this could prove to be something that's physically impossible. However, many couples not hampered by any physical obstacles find fisting can be an extremely pleasurable experience for both the woman and the man. Just to be clear, I'm specifically referring to the act of a man fisting a woman, although there are many couples out there who enjoy the exact opposite. The truth is when it comes to how to fist properly, it doesn't really matter whether it's you fisting your partner or your partner sticking her fist up your ass— there is a proper way to fist.

"Kinky is using a feather, perverted is using the whole chicken."
—Unknown

The Proper Way to Fist a Lady

1. You should wear a latex glove on your fisting hand. This will prevent you from gouging her pussy with your fingernails. It will also provide an all-around smooth surface for your hand, making insertion easier. An extra-large condom can serve in a pinch.
2. You should have plenty of her favorite lube on hand. Just make sure it's compatible with latex if you're wearing a glove or condom. As a rule of thumb, you should add lube every time you add another finger.
3. I have found that the missionary position is the best to use when introducing a woman to fisting. In this position, I have been most successful when I approach the pussy palm-up.
4. Now, starting palm-up, slowly insert your index finger, followed by your middle, ring, and pinkie. As you work your hand in, you'll need to overlap your middle finger with your index finger and your ring finger with your pinkie, and fold your thumb into your palm as shown.

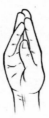

5. Okay, here comes the tricky part! Withdraw your four fingers to their tips and straighten out your thumb so it's resting in the index crease between your middle and ring fingers. (See illustration on the next page.)
6. You will now need to hold this hand position as you gradually start working it in. You will need to be especially careful as you try to push past your knuckles, which will be the widest part of your hand. Once past the knuckles, you should find it

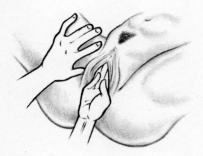

fairly easy to get wrist-deep. If you are finding it difficult to push past your knuckles, you can use your fingers (by spreading them out and retracting them back into position) to gently stretch her vaginal opening until she is able to accept you.

7. Once you've achieved wrist depth, you will need to carefully fold your thumb into your palm and slowly begin to ball your other four fingers over your thumb, into a fist.

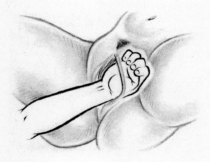

8. Once you have your hand balled into a fist, you should turn your fist over so that you are looking at the top of your wrist. This will provide a more natural motion for you and a more comfortable path for your fist to travel inside her. Now that you are in proper fisting position, you should start with slow movements and talk to her. As she lets you know she is getting more relaxed, you can start getting creative with your fist-pumping action, just as you would with your cock!

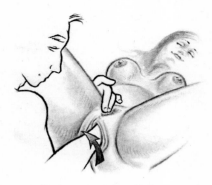

9. It is quite possible that the powerful contractions of her orgasm will cause her pussy muscles to create a vacuum seal around your fist. This can make withdrawal difficult. In order to break this seal, you can use a finger of your free hand and run it along the back of your "busy" hand until you are able to slide it into her pussy and gently pull upward, away from the back of your fist. Now, as you begin to slide your fist out of her pussy, slowly unfurl your fingers as you extract your hand.

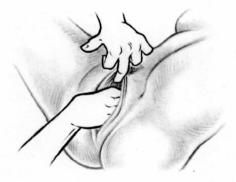

Fisting Odds and Ends

1. There is no such thing as a "fisting quickie." This is one of those games you better count on going well into extra innings before you start playing.

2. The first time a woman is fisted is an event much like losing her virginity, giving her first blow job, or getting fucked in the ass for the first time—you should treat it as such.

3. Giving her a vibrator to masturbate with, rubbing her clit with your free hand, or eating her out during the encounter will go a long way to helping her relax both mentally and vaginally, or anally, for that matter. Yes, there are women who enjoy a fist up the ass as well! However, they are the rarest of breeds and most definitely achieved a black belt in vaginal fisting before initially attempting the feat!

Throw Her a Breaking Ball

For some of you those "curveballs" might seem over-the-top or even outrageous. In this case, you might want to start off slower, or with "breaking balls," if you will. Those of you who hear complaints about not being affectionate, verbal, or romantic enough will find the following especially effective:

1. Hug her from behind and whisper sweet nothings in her ear.
2. Serve her breakfast in bed.
3. Surprise her on a nonspecial day with her favorite flowers or candy. (You should know her favorite!)
4. Tell her how good her ass looks in those pants.
5. Offer to scrub her back while she's taking a shower.
6. Take her for a walk on the beach.
7. Offer her a foot massage when she's had a rough day. (Do it right—use lotion or oil.)
8. Surprise her by taking her shopping for something specific like a new dress or a new pair of shoes. If you don't specify, you could end up spending more time and money than you'd like.
9. Tell her how pretty she looks.
10. Surprise her by picking up the chick flick that she was dying to see but there was no way in hell she was going to get you to see,

along with her favorite snack items—even if it means having to sit through *The Sisterhood of the Traveling Pants,* god help you!

These might seem like small gestures, but to a woman they can be seen as monumental milestones that are worthy of being noted in calendars and diaries. It really doesn't matter what pitch you throw; the key to becoming the ace of her mound is creativity and execution. Hey, if you've been developing a splitter and feel it's ready for the major leagues—by all means, throw it, man! Having said that, I do have to warn you against throwing "knucklehead" balls, which would cover both stupid and dangerous ideas. For example, a stupid idea would be to take a woman to the zoo and reveal your bestiality fantasies while telling her you have gone to great lengths to arrange for her to spend some sexy time with the park's newest attraction from China, Poon Tang the panda. An example of a dangerous idea would be choking. Some of you guys are into choking your partners during sex. Maybe you got the idea from a porno you watched or maybe your partner actually asked you to do it—but I'm here to tell you that if you're not careful, you can very easily find your ass being tried in a court of law for manslaughter. No joke, you can very easily kill your partner by choking her. Don't try telling me you know what you're doing either; that's what hundreds of guys say every year before they accidentally kill the women they are having sex with. In case this is all news to you, many men and women engage in this type of activity. It is technically called asphyxiophilia or erotic asphyxiation, and it involves depleting a person's oxygen supply to the brain, which produces a euphoric sensation along with an increase in adrenaline production; or in other words, it's supposed to make for more intense orgasms. The practice actually dates back to the early 1600s, when it was used as a treatment for erectile dysfunction after medical practitioners of the times noted that men would get hard while being hanged and would occasionally ejaculate during the hanging. While the practice was

Humans and dolphins are the only species that have sex for pleasure.

discontinued as an E.D. treatment, it continues being experimented with as a tool for sexual enhancement today. I say *don't do it*! It's not worth the risk involved when there are so many other ways to go about enhancing your sex! Shit, you should have a buttload of ideas from this book by now! And by the way, if any of you guys run into a woman who tells you about all the pleasure she can deliver by choking you while you come—keep running! Many men have died from asphyxiation, including Kichizo Ishida, a Japanese man who was accidently killed by his lover Sada Abe. After she discovered what she did, she proceeded to cut off his penis and testicles and carry them around in her purse for a few days, until her arrest. You don't want to end up like poor Kichizo, do you? It's one thing to be a knucklehead but it's a lot worse to be a dead knucklehead!

I feel safe assuming that you knew it was against the law to kill someone while having sex with them well before you picked up this book. I'll bet my sweet bippy, though, that you weren't aware of the following laws that still exist in the United States and throughout the world to this day:

- Sex toys are illegal in Alabama.
- Sleeping naked is illegal in Minnesota.
- Oral sex is illegal in Indiana.
- Anal intercourse is illegal in Cincinnati, Ohio.
- It is illegal in Minnesota for a man to have intercourse with a live fish.
- It is illegal to have sex in a graveyard in North Carolina.
- In Oblong, Illinois, it's illegal to have sex on your wedding day if you're hunting or fishing.
- It is illegal for a man to seduce a woman by promising to marry her in Mississippi.
- In Newcastle, Wyoming, it is illegal to have sex in a walk-in meat locker.
- It is illegal for a man to fire his gun when his lover reaches orgasm in Connorsville, Wisconsin.
- If you're arrested for soliciting a prostitute in Oklahoma, your name and picture will be shown on TV.
- In Washington, it is illegal for a man to have sex with any animal that weighs more than forty pounds.

- In Ames, Iowa, a husband may not take more than three gulps of beer while lying in bed with his wife.
- Flirting will get you thirty days in Little Rock, Arkansas.

Now, if you happen to live outside of the United States or are a frequent international traveler, you should be aware of the following:

- The penalty for masturbation in Indonesia is decapitation.
- In Santa Cruz, Bolivia, it is illegal for a man to have sex with a woman and her daughter at the same time.
- In Lebanon, men are legally allowed to have sex with female animals. Sex with male animals is punishable by death.
- In most Middle Eastern countries, it is a mortal sin to eat the flesh of a lamb after you've had intercourse with it.

Hey, don't look at me. I didn't write them. I just want you guys to be as well informed as possible, just in case you get any sudden urges to satisfy your curiosity about what it's like to make love to a male goat while you're vacationing in Lebanon. What can I say—I got your back!

CHAPTER 25

Three the Hard Way

rust me when I say there is no one more eager to tell you that a threesome with two women is the best thing since sliced bread. Yes, there are men who have had fantastic threesome experiences, and I count myself as one of them, but they are just too few and far between for me to be able to recommend it without yelling out a few words of caution.

I place the blame on two culprits: love and jealousy. Love tends to complicate things when a third wheel is introduced into an intimate relationship, leading to jealousy. And I'm not only referring to the female partner becoming jealous, although this is very common; I'm also talking about the man becoming jealous of the intimate bond that forms between the two ladies. The fact is most people, man or woman, are not emotionally prepared to see someone they love having sex with someone else! Of course, the rub is that you'll never really know until you give it a go. Yet, if you give it a go and it goes all wrong, you could do irreparable damage to the relationship you're in.

For example, take the story of Jason and Monica, a couple that I met at a swing party on New Year's Eve 1991. Jason had been pressuring Monica to participate in a three-way with another woman for the last year of their nearly three-year-old relationship. Jason finally got Monica to cave by agreeing to a threesome with another man at a later date. As Jason told it, he "called her bluff"—thinking she wouldn't have the guts to go through it. Fast-forward to New Year's Eve, one of the biggest swinging nights of the year; Jason and Monica were at a swing party sponsored by the largest swingers' association in the United States. The way these parties work is everybody gets together in the ballroom of a hotel for mingling, drinking, dancing, and a fair share of groping. This is when the after-party deals are made, and you'll hear things like:

"You wanna swap wives?"

"We're looking for a third."

"My wife wants to be gangbanged."

"I just wanna watch my wife get fucked!"

"We're looking for one more couple for the orgy in suite 1682."

Jason and Monica ended up at the orgy in suite 1682. There were fourteen other couples in the room plus a few single women—my girlfriend Cristi and I were in attendance as well. As a matter of fact, I was smoking a joint with Monica and a few others when Jason walked up with a pretty blonde on his arm and introduced her to Monica. They all had a short conversation, Monica asked for one last hit, and the three of them disappeared from sight. From that point, things get slightly blurry for me, as I proceeded to have sex with four different women that night and two others took turns tossing my salad. Needless to say, it was a good night for me!

I can't say the same for Jason. Jason, Monica, and the blonde lay themselves out in a corner of the large "common area" and started going at it. I imagine Jason was enjoying himself immensely at this point, maybe a bit too much. I am told that Jason started off by having sex with the blonde, lost control, and came within the first five minutes—leaving him unable to take care of Monica. Of course, Monica got pissed and told Jason she was going to smoke a cigarette. Fast-forward fifteen to twenty minutes later; one of the bedrooms had drawn a crowd, and since I was taking a break at the time, I moseyed on over to check things out. Yes, it was Monica, screaming, as a huge black cock slammed into her from behind! Just when Monica yelled, "Oh my fucking god, I've never come so hard in my life," I noticed Jason pushing through the doorway, and this is what followed:

Jason: You stupid fuckin' bitch! What the fuck are you doing? You're fucking a nigger?

Black Dude: What the fuck you say? [still pumping his dick in and out of Monica, only slower]

Jason: I wasn't talking to you.

Black Dude: [as he pulls his anaconda out of Monica] Well, I'm
    talking to you!

Then the black dude started whaling on Jason and things got chaotic
as Jason bled profusely from his nose and mouth. All I know is that Monica was still fucking the black dude forty-five minutes later. A few months
after the incident, I heard that Jason ended up needing facial reconstruc-
tion surgery and Monica ended up moving in with the black dude and
his girlfriend—to form what is referred to as a triad relationship, or a
permanent threesome, if you will. I guess Monica was into threesomes
after all.

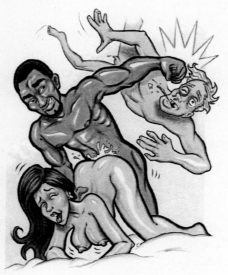

To summarize this cautionary tale, if you and your partner are in love
and are contemplating having a threesome, I say don't do it! It's just not
worth it when you weigh risk versus reward. On the other hand, if you
have a female fuck friend who is up for the experience, by all means proceed full steam ahead. You really don't have anything to lose, except for a
few teeth, I suppose. No matter which category you fall into, let me give
you a few pointers to help the experience match the fantasy as closely as
possible.

Animal Testing—Spend a night at a strip club with your partner. While strip clubs are a good place to meet women who would be interested in threesome propositions, that is not the purpose of this expedition. During your visit, you want to get as many beavers, pussies, and asses rubbing all over you and your partner as you can afford. This will be a good test of the jealous impulses for both of you and will give you a good idea if you should proceed with the pursuit of this particular fantasy.

If you both pass that test, the next thing to consider is how to go about finding the right third. Whatever you do, don't even think about doing it with anyone either of you already knows. That's just a recipe for disaster. No, you need to find someone neither of you have ever met before, so you're both starting off on an even playing field. There are three ways to go about finding a willing woman.

Swinger/Adult Dating Web sites—They are easily found on the Internet and can provide a safe, nonintimidating arena in which you can ease yourselves into the scene. These sites are also advantageous because of the quantity and variety of potential thirds you have to choose from.

Swing Parties/Sex Clubs—There is a huge swinging community out there and they're not just swinging in their homes. There are many sex clubs located throughout the United States—throughout the world, for that matter. And there are swingers' events sponsored by large organizations going on throughout the year. Seek and ye shall find.

Strip Clubs/Prostitutes—I know, I'm going to get some shit for lumping them together. I am not saying that all strippers are prostitutes, nor that it would be a bad thing if they were. I am saying, from personal experience, that there are more than a few strippers who are willing to sell more than a lap dance. The point is that a strip club is an excellent place to meet

"Sex between a man and woman can be absolutely wonderful—provided you get between the right man and the right woman."
—Woody Allen

women who are more likely to consider your proposal than, say, a woman you meet at a bar or a supermarket. Whether or not they will consider taking you up on the proposal for free is a whole other story. Of course, we know the prostitute isn't doing anything for free! The fact that she's a pro could go a long way toward easing any jealousies that could potentially arise. Plus, her experience should be a bonus that makes the experience more pleasurable for both of you.

Wherever you decide to go "hunting," you should let your female partner have the final say in the decision as to who to finally approach. Again, letting her have control over the third will help tame the jealous beast that might lurk inside her.

Once you have decided upon your third, you're obviously on your way to fulfilling your fantasy. I do want to suggest a few more things for you to keep in mind.

Establish Rules—Many couples who swing find it helpful to establish a set of rules for each other before these types of alternate sexual encounters. These rules should be mutually agreed upon and discussed well in advance of any encounter. Here are a few of the more common rules that I know of couples having:

> No kissing the third.
> Each must never leave the other alone during encounters.
> Male must orgasm inside partner.
> Always use condoms.
> No oral sex.
> No anal sex.

Hey, I didn't make up those rules, but I'm sure each couple had their own reasoning behind each one of them. The important thing is to establish a set of rules that you are both comfortable with, and follow them.

Divide Your Attention Evenly—Actually, I'd take it even a step further and make sure you pay slightly more attention to your partner, just to be on the safe side.

Stay Connected During the Sex—Always try to stay in touch with your partner in some way while you are having sex with the third. Take a gander at the illustrations below to see what I mean:

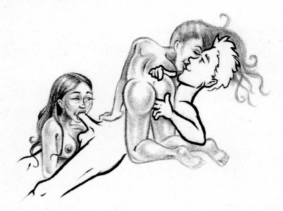

If the third is giving you head, you can position your partner so you can play with her pussy and ass.

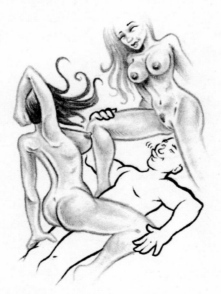

If the third is on top of you, why not invite your partner to sit on your face?

Careful Reflection—While it is natural, healthy, and stimulating to discuss the experience with your partner after the fact, you should avoid centering the discussion on the third and instead focus on the group moments or the girl/girl action between your partner and your guest.

The Other Threesome

This is certainly a much easier fantasy to pursue. I mean, it really doesn't matter what your partner looks like, you'll have no trouble finding a guy willing to fuck her. But is this a risk you really want to take? Have you really thought about the potential consequences of initiating this type of activity? Whether you think you have or not, I'm gonna lay it out to you for my peace of mind.

- How will you feel if you can't get it up but the third wheel can, leaving you to watch your partner getting her world rocked all night long?
- How will you feel if the third wheel has a bigger cock than you?
- How will you feel if your partner has an orgasm with the third wheel but not you?
- How will you feel if your partner asks you to invite the third wheel over again?

You seriously need to think about these things if you're contemplating sharing your partner with another man. Only couples with the tightest and most intimate bonds can thrive while engaging in these types of alternative sexual behaviors. As with the other scenario discussed here, my advice is to leave it be. A well-placed dildo along with some dirty talk can go a long way toward simulating the fantasy for both of you.

Now, in an effort to make things even easier for you, here is a list of

"Jealousy is all the fun you think they had."—Erica Jong

"How many of our daydreams would darken into nightmares, were there a danger of their coming true!"
—Logan Pearsall Smith

swinging-related US sites that will provide you with a host of resources to explore:

SWINGER ORGANIZATIONS
Nasca.com (Northern American Swing Club Association)

MEET OTHER SWINGERS
Tfexp.com (The Friendship Express)
Connectionmag.com
Swingerdatelink.com

TRAVEL FOR SWINGERS
Ipcresorts.com
Hedonism.com
Desire-resorts.com

PORTAL FOR SWINGERS
Playcouples.com

CHAPTER 26

Cherry Picking

Man will travel the globe and in some cases risk his freedom in quest of the rarest of all female flowers—the virgin. Personally, I don't get it and find virgin sex appeal to be more urban legend than anything. It seems to me that having sex with a woman who most likely has no idea what she's doing is like going for a ride in a race car with a driver who has never driven a stick shift: It just doesn't sound like a lot of fun. I do know that if I walked into a sex therapist's office and confessed a preference for virgins, I would be asked to answer questions like these:

Do you think your preference for sex with virgins has to do with feelings of insecurity you have about the size of your penis or quality of your sexual performance, as a virgin would have nothing to compare you to?

Do you think your preference for sex with virgins has to do with a fear or prior experience you've had with sexually transmitted disease and your feeling that "virgin sex" is safer?

Do you think your preference for sex with virgins stems from an attraction you have to younger girls? If so, is it possible you've developed or are developing an unhealthy attraction to underage girls?

I treat the subject seriously because women take their virginity very seriously. Unless she's drunk or impaired in some way, a woman is not likely to give it up to just any guy. It's going to be a guy she has strong feelings for, at the least! And knowingly taking a woman's virginity while she's drunk or impaired is a risky proposition and a sign of bad judgment on the man's part.

I believe a man who has the opportunity to be a woman's first needs to accept the added responsibility that is inherent in the "honor." Most importantly, the man doing the deflowering should not be doing so under false pretenses. That is, the man has to be honest in expressing how he feels about the woman. Let's face it, there are some men who will say anything it takes to get laid, whether they actually mean it or not. They have the unique ability to manipulate women with words. But those games are best played with women who are more experienced and already at the point of playing similar games themselves.

A negative first-time experience can be absolutely devastating to a woman. In addition to the heartache and mental anguish, it could also cause a loss of self-esteem and/or feelings of depression. In other words, a negative first-time experience can really fuck with a woman's head!

Now that I've hopefully pounded that into yours, I think you'll find the pounding well worth it—as I am about to let you in on the secrets to successfully deflowering a virgin that have been passed from generation to generation in my family for the last five centuries. The secrets were written on a scroll that was found by a slave working on building the Great Wall of China back in the sixteenth century. My greatest of all grandfathers, Irving Glasser, had a bagel stand near the Great Wall at the time and was offered the scroll

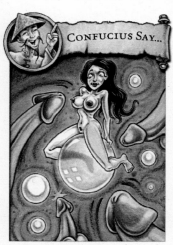

Virginity like bubble—
one prick all gone

by the slave as payment for a bagel with extra cream cheese. Irv accepted because he felt sorry for the hungry fellow; he had no idea of the secrets that were contained on the scroll until he was able to have the ancient writing translated. Here is what it said . . .

The man who try to pluck flower
from unplowed field, need two
things for success . . .
Plenty of lube
and
a shitload of patience!

In all seriousness, though, there are a few things you can do to ensure the best possible experience for you both:

Choose a Romantic Setting/Create a Romantic Atmosphere—I guess I'm trying to say that the backseat of your 1973 Pinto is probably not the best place for a proper deflowering. Aside from that, I can promise you that any efforts you make to add a touch of romance to the encounter will be more than appreciated by her!

The Sweet Stuff—Considering this is her first time, a monumental event in any woman's life, she is likely to be nervous and unsure of herself. You can go a long way toward providing the comfort and reassurance she needs by showering her with kisses, supplying lots of foreplay, maintaining eye contact, and whispering plenty of sweet nothings into her ear.

Since this is her first experience, there are probably a few things to avoid as well:

1. **Watch Your Mouth**—It's probably best to keep your words on the soft and sweet side of the fence as opposed to the "Suck it, bitch!" approach. Get too crude with a first-timer and you risk the possibility that the only thing you'll be sticking anywhere is your foot in your own mouth!
2. **No Gymnastics**—The first time is probably not the best time to start flipping her around like a Raggedy Ann doll. Keep it simple, stupid! One or two positions maximum should do the trick, as it's about making her feel like a princess at an opera instead of a porn star in a mosh pit! Besides, if you break her off something proper that first time, you should have plenty of opportunities to expose her to your entire bag of tricks in the future.

3. **Don't Be an Ostrich**—Try to avoid your natural instinct to bury your head in the pillow and jackhammer away at her. Again, you need to focus on maintaining eye contact when you're not kissing her.

4. **No Butts About It**—If you haven't explored her ass up to this point, the first time is probably not the best time to begin your anal explorations.

Seriously, it's really a matter of common sense, isn't it? Go slow, take your time, be gentle, have fun, warm her up right, plenty of lube, shitload of patience, etc., etc.

Finally, I want to take a moment to consider the question "Where do I find a virgin?" My answer: "Hell if I know!" Like I said, I've never had much of an appetite for virgins—and I didn't have much luck finding a better answer to this question while doing my research. Unless, that is, you are looking for a college-aged virgin. For you, I have found what could be very useful information. This chart shows the results of a survey conducted by *Counterpoint* magazine at Wellesley College in the US. It depicts the virginity rates among students according to the student's major:

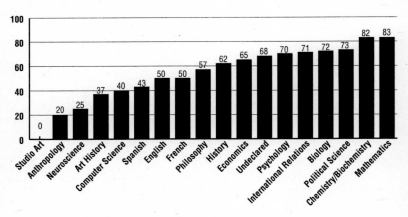

Percent of students that are virgins, by Wellesley major

Twenty-nine percent of us are virgins when we marry.

It seems quite clear that the chemistry and mathematics departments are the places to start. If I was interested enough in the pursuit of purity, I might take some hints from the chart and assume women who have jobs related to the majors with the highest virginity rates, i.e., accountants, chemists, and doctors, are my best bets. I would also suggest attending social functions sponsored by religious organizations. Conversely, looking for a virgin in the US at a strip club, bar, nightclub, art gallery, Alcoholics Anonymous meeting, or for that matter in the entire states of New York, New Jersey, Florida, Illinois, Michigan, Ohio, Texas, California, Oregon, and Hawaii is like looking for a shard of class in any of the stars of *The Real Housewives of New Jersey*. Of course, you could always elect to go for the sure thing. While doing my research, I came across a young woman who was actually auctioning off her hymen. In this case, all you need is around $4,000,000, as the high bid was at $3,700,000 last time I checked.

"Virginity is the ideal of those who want to deflower."
—Karl Kraus

CHAPTER 27

Sex Toy Story

Introducing Her to Sex Toys

Knowing how and when to introduce your partner to sex toys can be a tricky proposition, especially if your partner happens to be of a conservative nature. And I think it's safe to assume that if you are the one doing the introducing, your partner is either very conservative or a very recently converted virgin. Of course, you could be involved with a woman who has prior experience with sex toys—just not with you—and you would like to introduce them into the relationship. Whichever is the case, it doesn't affect the advice I'm about to give you, as all those situations call for similar knowledge and action. Now, unless you're going to be giving her a vibrator as a birthday or Christmas gift, I suggest that you try to do the shopping with her. In addition to it being an intimate bonding experience, you will turn her on with your display of dildo expertise! If you do take her shopping, make sure you take her to one of those new adult stores that are light and bright as opposed to one of those seedy holes-in-the-wall that smell like they've been marinated in fermented semen.

Since we are using the word "introducing," I believe it is best to start off slow, so to speak. In other words, buying her a ten-inch rubber penis with pulsating purple veins probably isn't a good choice. Instead, there are many products available that will deliver the goods but are much less visually intimidating. On the following pages you will find the types of sex toys I recommend for beginners. You'll have to decide exactly which one(s) fit your needs best . . .

The Rabbit—This is one of the most popular vibrators ever made! If your partner is a fan of *Sex and the City,* she'll recognize this as Miranda's favorite. In any case, this battery-operated product actually looks like a rabbit's head, as opposed to a penis, and has a small anal tickler attached as well.

Pocket Rocket—This is a very small yet very powerful battery-operated vibrator that is not only excellent for her to masturbate with but is also perfect for integrating into your sex play!

Back Massagers—These may be big and clumsy but they'll certainly do the trick for her. Much better for masturbation than incorporating into sex play because of the size and electric cord, these products can be purchased in many "mainstream" outlets, which can alleviate the worry of potential embarrassment from visiting an adult store or Web site. You'll find there are many different "back massagers" to choose from. I would recommend the Hitachi Magic Wand as it seems to do the trick for many of my hot female Twitter friends.

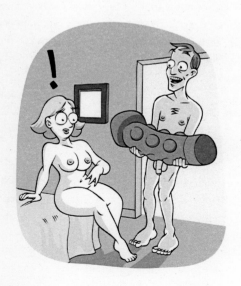

"The best sex I ever had was with my vibrator."—Eva Longoria

Slim Line—These battery-operated toys are shaped like a penis without the detail and are excellent for both clitoral and internal stimulation, as well as both masturbation and use during "sexy time."

Smooth Contour—I consider these to be among the new generation of sex toys. They are designed specifically with the more conservative woman in mind. Simply put, they just don't look like sex toys but they sure act like them.

Eco-Friendly—Even if your partner is a tree-hugger, there are now products made especially for her. Whether it's glass, wood, or silicone, you can find the perfect sex toy for your ecocentric girl.

Other Unique Products You Should Know About

Kegelmaster—This is not actually a toy but a "pussy exerciser." By using this, your partner will not only strengthen her PC (pubococcygeus) muscles, which will enable quicker, more intense orgasms, but it will also make her pussy feel tighter to you. Products like ben wa balls or smart balls are designed to produce similar results.

Remote-Control Bullet—Like vibrating panties, this product can be used during a night out on the town or in the confines of the bedroom. Great for clitoral, vaginal, or anal stimulation.

Eroscillator—It might look like an electric toothbrush but it won't help whiten her smile. It *will* induce tartar-shattering orgasms from her, though. The Eroscillator is specifically designed for clitoral stimulation. This thing will deliver her a lot of bang for your buck.

Love Swing—This is more of something for both of you to enjoy. If anything, it gets you out of the bed. I've used them in quite a few of my movies and always received inquiries from women asking where they can purchase a swing. They do require some setup but the effort is well worth it!

Sybian—This is probably the most expensive and most powerful vibrator available today. It has a saddle-like hump design that the woman straddles as she sits on it. It has multispeed vibration and rotational controls that allow for clitoral and G-spot stimulation.

G-spot Toys—Aside from the Sybian, there are many less expensive yet very effective toys specifically designed to stimulate the G-spot. These will all feature some degree of curvature at the top or head of the toy. They can be found in almost every material—including metal, glass, rubber, wood, and plastic—depending on your preference.

Anal Toys—In addition to the graduated butt plugs that I recommended to you in chapter 22, there are quite a few choices when it comes to anal-oriented toys. Mirna happens to love anal beads. Whether they are the kind that vibrate or not doesn't really matter—she just loves it when they are slowly pulled out of her ass as she is orgasming.

We-Vibe—This is another of those next-generation products that is becoming known for its unique design, stimulation versatility, and the rave reviews it is getting from women!

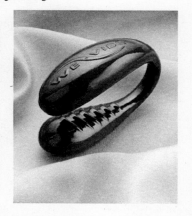

Fingertip Vibrators—These are small, powerful vibrators that you actually wear on your fingertips. These are excellent for use during sex!

Vibrating Cock Ring—Another product designed for both of you to enjoy. This is slipped around the base of your cock and will help you maintain your erection by not allowing blood to flow out of your penis. It will also buzz her clit on every downstroke and make you both feel as if you have a vibrating erection.

Vibrating Tongue Rings/Studs—Yup, that's right. For you guys with pierced tongues this might be a way to pleasantly surprise her the next time you're dining down south. Of course, if your partner has a pierced tongue, this could be the perfect gift for both of you.

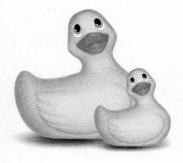

I Rub My Duckie—She'll wanna fuck after she warms herself up in the bathtub with one of these waterproof, battery-operated duckies. She will not only think it's adorable, but you might find her taking a lot more baths as well!

Liberator Wedge—As I mentioned in the chapter 21, incorporating a pillow into your sex play can be helpful in positioning your partner so that you have more direct contact with her G-spot. Now there are companies that make pillows specifically for this purpose—like this product from Liberator.

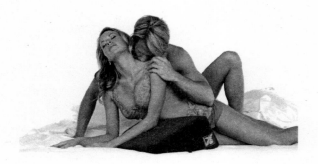

Sportsheets—This is an excellent product for those of you who have an interest in getting involved with bondage, discipline, and the like. Basically, this is a set containing soft Velcro bedsheets along with Velcro wrist and ankle restraints. All you do is slip the bedsheet over your mattress, place the restraints on your partner, and then just "stick" her to the bed in any desirable position.

EARLY SEX TOY SKETCHES MEANT FOR APPROVAL BY KING GEORGE II

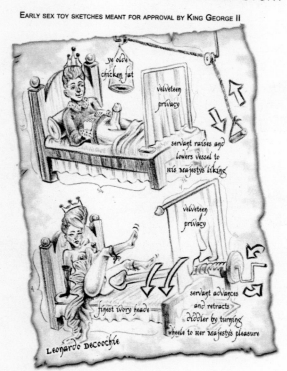

What About Us Guys?

There are many products out there that are designed specifically for men. These would include cock rings, prostate stimulators, and masturbatory devices. Since I've already mentioned cock rings, I'm going to focus on the latter two.

Prostate Stimulators—These have become very popular over the last decade, which has led to an abundance of these products being available today. In my opinion, there are two companies that excel in this area—Nexus and Aneros. They might be slightly pricey but their designs and functionality are second to none.

Masturbatory Devices—Again, there are literally thousands of products designed to enhance masturbation, from life-size silicone females with

According to the Museum of Sex, the vibrator was originally introduced as a medicinal treatment for female "hysteria" during the nineteenth century. The resulting orgasms helped doctors dissipate hysteria's anxiety-related symptoms.

It is estimated that between 20 and 30 percent of adults have used sex toys at least once in their lives.

vibrating anuses to a pussy you can carry in your pocket. My favorite are the masturbation cylinders made by Fleshjack. These are realistic, flesh-like female body parts that are actually cock sleeves. They are made to resemble a mouth, pussy, or ass and are contained within something similar to a Slurpee cup with a screw-on cap. Anyway, you fuck it and it almost feels like the real thing . . . almost!

The Blowguard—This product, developed by a dentist, turns your partner's mouth into a living, breathing vibrating orifice.

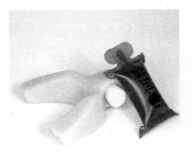

Other Things You Should Know

When buying a sex toy with a motor, you should know that toys with motors built in the USA or Japan are generally superior to those built in China and Taiwan.

If you are buying a sex toy made of soft rubber or jelly, you should always look for products that are phthalate-free. Phthalates are a family of chemicals that are used to soften hard plastics and rubbers to give them that squishy feel. These chemicals are now considered to be toxic and have been linked to cervical cancer.

Buyer Beware

While it is not officially recognized by the medical community as an addiction, some women can become very attached to their favorite vibrator. For the woman, there really is no problem . . . as long as she can afford the batteries and electric bills. The potential problem falls directly in our laps. A woman who overindulges can raise her stimulation/orgasm thresholds beyond that which any man without an "S" stamped on his chest could match. A situation like this could prove frustrating for any man unless he's willing to do one of two things:

Accept the fact that you are part of a triad relationship and extend an open invitation for all future sexual encounters to her vibrator.
   OR

Invented around 500 A.D., ben wa balls were originally used to increase men's pleasure during intercourse. A single ball would be placed into the vagina before the man inserted his penis. The ball was said to increase sensation and friction for the man. Later, the balls were paired and used by women to increase the strength of their pelvic floor muscles.

The first cock rings were made in China from the eyelids of goats with eyelashes intact. The eyelids were tied around the man's erection, and the lashes were said to tickle the balls.

Speak to her openly and honestly about your concerns and suggest she go cold-turkey and abstain from all vibe usage for a substantial period of time—at least six to eight weeks. She will have regained all or most of her natural sensitivity during this time, after which you can reintroduce her to vibrators during your sex play on "special occasions" and ask her to masturbate with energy-eating devices in moderation. She can go to town with her fingers, any non-motorized dildo, a hairbrush, the eraser tip of a pencil, a toothbrush, a high-heeled shoe, her favorite stuffed animal or pillow, a beer bottle, a cucumber, frozen hot dogs, a koosh ball, etc, etc, etc.

CHAPTER 28

Peep Show

As far as women and pornography go, times have changed. Many more women are accepting of adult movies compared to just a decade ago. The issue most women have with adult content is with the way it's presented, or the context, if you will, as opposed to the adult nature of the content itself. In fact, I would take it a step further and say many women enjoy hard-core materials as much as men, as long as it's the right type of hard-core material. Women are looking for things most of us guys don't think twice about. Here are some of the elements you should look for when choosing an X-rated movie that both you and your partner can enjoy:

Most women prefer a little story line to go along with their oral, anal, and vaginal sex.

Most women prefer the depiction of consensual sex and the girls receiving pleasure as opposed to them being portrayed as "sperm receptacles."

Most women want to see attractive participants, especially the male performers.

Hot sex in exotic locations seems to be a winning combination for female viewers.

Most women will be receptive to adult movies that have educational value.

Spoofs of or tributes to popular mainstream titles are appealing to women because of the familiarity factor.

A touch of comedy will go a long way toward helping woman relax and "get loose" during the viewing.

With those elements in mind, I've taken the opportunity to put together a list of some of the best female-friendly adult movies for your consideration:

TITLE STUDIO (Year Released) DIRECTOR	CAST	GENRE
Amanda by Night Caballero Home Video (1981) Robert McCallum	Veronica Hart, Mai Lin, Jamie Gillis, Ron Jeremy, Don Fernando, Eric Edwards, Samantha Fox, Michael Morrison, Lisa De Leeuw, Jon Martin, Arcadia Lake, R. Bolla, Frank Hollowell, Herschel Savage, Pat Manning, Brooke West, Nicole Noir, Lee Carroll	Drama
Bliss VCA (1999) Antonio Passolini	Juli Ashton, Tina Tyler, Gina Ryder, Nikita, Chloe, Steve Hatcher, Tony Tedeschi, Joel Lawrence	Romance
Conquest Wicked Pictures (1996) Brad Armstrong, Greg Steel	Asia Carrera, Tom Byron, Vince Voyeur, Missy, Kia, Alex Sanders, Mark Davis, Juli Ashton, Shayla LaVeaux, Sahara Sands, Brad Armstrong, Julie Rage, Claudio, Jenna Jameson, Alex Dane, Sean Rider	Drama
Debbie Does Dallas VCX (1978) Jim Clark	Eric Edwards, Merle Michaels, Christie Ford, Bambi Woods, David Morris, Arcadia Lake, Rikki O'Neal, Georgette Sanders, R. Bolla, Herschel Savage, Jake Teague, Robin Byrd, David Pierce, Kasey Rodgers, Ben Pierce, Tony Mansfield, Jenny Cole, Paul Hughs, Peter Lerman, Debbie Lewis, Steve Marshall	Comedy
Fade to Black CDI Home Video (1988) Ron Jeremy	Kascha, Lauryl Canyon, Nina DePonca, Ona Z, Tiffany Storm, Darryl Edwards, Francois, Ray Victory, Stewart Harris, Tom Byron	Drama

TITLE STUDIO (Year Released) DIRECTOR	CAST	GENRE
Fallen Wicked Pictures (2008) Brad Armstrong	Randy Spears, Brad Armstrong, Tommy Gunn, Jessica Drake, Niko, Shyla Stylez, Barrett Blade, Jenaveve Jolie, Angie Savage, Marcus London, Barry Scott, Derrick Pierce, Alektra Blue, Lana Croft, Jenna Haze, Ryder Skye, Michelle McLaren, Jada Fire, Hunter Bryce, Eric Masterson, Herschel Savage, Randy Spears, Jennifer Dark, Gianna Lynn,	Drama
Female Ejaculation: A Complete Guide Seymore Butts Home Movies (2003) Seymore Butts	Alisha Klass, Tina Cherry, Montana Gunn, Lori Rivers, Taylor Hayes, Allison Embers, Jewel Valmont, Bonita Saint, Mary Jane, Jordan McKnight, Taren Steel, Seymore Butts.	Instructional
Flashpoint Wicked Pictures (1997) Brad Armstrong	Jenna Jameson, Asia Carrera, Jill Kelly, Sydnee Steele, Veronica Hart, Sindee Coxx, Brittany Andrews, Missy, Johnni Black, T. T. Boy, Eric Price, Mike Horner, Brad Armstrong, Steve Drake, Jonathan Morgan, Mickey G	Action/ Adventure
Hidden Obsessions Ultimate Video (1992) Andrew Blake	Celeste, Deidre Holland, Dominique Simone, Francesca Le, Heather Hart, Janine, Julia Ann, Kym Wilde, Lauryl Canyon, Marissa Malibu, Melanie Moore, P. J. Sparxx, Paula Price, Sheila Stone, Skye Blue, Sunset Thomas, Tracy West, Jon Dough, Marc Wallice, Nick East, Peter North, Randy West, Steve Drake, Woody Long	Fantasy
How to Eat Pussy Like a Champ Seymore Butts Home Movies (2008) Seymore Butts	Mari Possa, Kenzie Marie, Nina Hartley, Kimber Lace, Morgan Reigns, Rucca Page, Sunny Lane, Veronica Rayne, Jack Lawrence, Ron Jeremy, Seymore Butts	Instructional
Insatiable 1 Caballero Home Video (1980) Godfrey Daniels	Marilyn Chambers, John Holmes, John Leslie, Jessie St. James, Serena, David Morris, Richard Pacheco, Mike Ranger	Drama

continued

TITLE STUDIO (Year Released) DIRECTOR	CAST	GENRE
Island Fever 1 Digital Playground (2000) Joone	Bobby Vitale, Julia Ann, Tera Patrick, Devin Wolf, Briana Banks	Fantasy
Jamaican Me Horny Seymore Butts Home Movies (2003) Seymore Butts	Mari Possa, Flower, Seymore Butts, Steven St. Croix, Herschel Savage	Gonzo
Night of the Giving Head Rodnievision (2008) Rodney Moore	Amber Rayne, Caroline Pierce, Claire Dames, Kylee Reese, Nikki Coxxx, Rucca Page, Samantha Sin, Veronica Rayne, Alan Stafford, Barry Scott, Brad Hardy, Chris Johnson, Christian XXX, Jack Vegas, Jarod Diamond, Mark Zane, Scott Lyons	Horror Spoof
Night Trips Caballero Home Video (1989) Andrew Blake	Jamie Summers, Porshe Lynn, Tanya DeVries, Tori Welles, Victoria Paris, Randy Spears, Ray Victory, Mark DeBruin, Peter North	Fantasy
Not Bewitched XXX Adam & Eve (2008) Will Ryder	Aurora Snow, Daisy Layne, Eva Angelina, Jenna Haze, Candice Nicole, Kelly Skyline, Madison Ivy, Marli Jane, Michelle Avanti, Nina Hartley, Sasha Grey, Sunny Lane, Teagan Presley, Winter Sky, Aaron Wilcox, Dane Cross, James Deen, Mike Horner, Nathan Threat	Comedy Spoof
Not the Bradys XXX Hustler Video (2006) Will Ryder	Jasmine Byrne, Mikey Butders, Leah Luv, Kurt Lockwood, Aurora Snow, Tee Reel, Paulina James, Veronique Vega, James Deen, Alana Evans, Mike Horner, Hillary Scott, Benjamin Brat	Comedy Spoof
Nothing to Hide Metro (1981) Anthony Spinelli	John Leslie, Erica Boyer, Misty Regan, Raven Turner, Holly McCall, Richard Pacheco, Tigr, Elizabeth Randolph, Jack Hoffey, Tom Ramar, Roy Phipps, Arianne, Katherine Remy, Ronald Gregg, Nicole Adams	Drama

TITLE STUDIO (Year Released) DIRECTOR	CAST	GENRE
Operation Desert Stormy Wicked Pictures (2007) Stormy Daniels	Stormy Daniels, Audrey Bitoni, Austin Kincaid, Eva Angelina, Jenna Haze, Kaylani Lei, Lorena Sanchez, Melissa Lauren, Nakita Kash, Nicole Sheridan, Roxy DeVille, Veronica Rayne, Marcus London, Randy Spears, Ron Jeremy, Steven St. Croix, Tommy Gunn, Tony De Sergio, Voodoo	Action/ Adventure
Pirates II: Stagnetti's Revenge Digital Playground (2008) Joone	Abbey Brooks, Belladonna, Brea Lynn, Brianna Love, Gabrielle Fox, Jenna Haze, Jesse Jane, Katsuni, Rhylee Richards, Riley Steele, Sasha Grey, Shawna Lenee, Shay Jordan, Shyla Stylez, Stoya, Veronica Rayne	Action/ Adventure
Space Nuts Wicked Pictures (2003) Jonathan Morgan	Stormy Daniels, Jessica Drake, Devinn Lane, Steve Hatcher, Julian, Kyle Stone, Evan Stone, Randy Spears, Phyllisha Anne, Kim Chambers, Scott Styles, Katie Morgan, Trevor Zen, Casey Pink, Amber Rain, Kaylani Lei, Hollie Stevens	Comedy Spoof
Tushy Tahitian Style Seymore Butts Home Movies (1998) Seymore Butts	Alexandra Nice, Alisha Klass, Samantha Stylle, Seymore Butts, Tom Byron	Gonzo
Xana and Dax: When Opposites Attract Comstock Films (2005) Tony Comstock	Xana, Dax	Romance
Night Trips: A Dark Odyssey Studio A Entertainment (2008) Andrew Blake	Charlotte Stokely, Kelly Summer, Kira Kane, Natasha Nice, Paola Rey, Sophia Santi, Aaron Wilcox, Eric Swiss, Essi X, Otto Bauer	Fantasy

Buyer Beware

There are many men, and women for that matter, who will tell you they are addicted to pornography. Whether or not this is truly an addiction, or a compulsion as I suspect, I have no doubt that excessive viewing of adult materials has done more than its fair share of damage to many individuals and/or relationships. Certainly the line between addictive or compulsive viewing habits and "normal" viewing habits is not black and white, but I can provide a few questions one may ask one's self if they were in doubt of whether or not they had "crossed the line":

1. Do you view pornography to deal with, deny, or avoid problems in your life?
2. Do you feel guilty or shameful after watching porn?

It is estimated that adult videos generate $20 billion in worldwide revenue each year.

The adult industry generates more revenue yearly than the US National Football League (NFL), National Basketball Association (NBA), Major League Baseball (MLB), and the National Hockey League (NHL) combined.

Twelve percent of all Web sites on the Internet display adult materials.

One out of three visitors to adult Web sites are women.

"My reaction to porn films is as follows: After the first ten minutes, I want to go home and screw. After the first twenty minutes, I never want to screw again as long as I live."
—Erica Jong

Seventeen percent of all women struggle with a pornography addiction.

3. Have you ever promised yourself that you would never watch porn again and subsequently broken the promise?
4. Do you spend more money than you can afford on pornographic materials?
5. Have you been accused of watching too much porn by a partner, friend, or family member?
6. Do you find yourself choosing to watch porn instead of initiating sex with your partner?
7. Do you fail to carry out responsibilities or meet commitments because of the time you spend watching porn?

Now, if someone were to tell me they answered yes to two or more of these questions, I would tell that person they need to seriously consider the depth of their involvement with pornographic materials and possibly go cold-turkey for a period of time in order to re-establish their control over the situation. If you or someone you know struggles with this problem there are many online resources offering information and support, including Pornaddictioninfo.com, No-porn.com, Newlifehabits.com, Xxxchurch.com, and Sexualrecovery.com.

Twenty-five percent of daily search engine requests (about 68,000,000 searches per day) are adult related.

CHAPTER 29

Infection Section

Once upon a time, I discovered I had genital warts. Actually I didn't know that I had genital warts at first. I just knew that there was a cluster of ugly-looking bumps on my cock—and I was fairly sure they shouldn't have been there! Even though this happened over twenty years ago, I am positive this discovery of mine happened in the month of March. I know this because I can remember becoming alarmed about the spring break trip to Palm Springs that was only three weeks away. After all, the whole purpose was to get laid, and I thought the cauliflower growing on my dick might not go over too well with the ladies! I was so concerned that I mentioned my discovery to my buddy Kurt that same night. I was amazed and, to be honest, somewhat relieved to find out he had made a similar discovery. We put our detective hats on and figured if we caught the same shit at the same time and hadn't fucked each other, then we must have caught it from the same girl at the same time. And only one girl matched that scenario: Tanya, the girl we gangbanged with eight of our other friends! It took us about a day to get in contact with all eight of them—some had already made the discovery and others examined themselves at our urging. All eight of them had contracted the speed bumps. Considering nine out of ten of us were all going to Palm Springs, we had a big problem that we needed to solve in less than three weeks! None of us wanted to tell our parents (we were all under eighteen at the time) and few of us had any money to spare for a doctor if we were going to make the trip. We hatched a plan to send a couple of us to the free clinic to see what we had and how it was treated. Once we had the pertinent info, we would all decide as a group how to proceed. Kurt and I volunteered to make the trip and left right after school the next day. This was the first free clinic either of us had ever been to and it lived up to all my expectations, or lack thereof. I was kinda nervous, fearing the worst possible diagnosis, although I had no idea what that might be.

After about thirty-five minutes of watching the news in the waiting room, I was the first called into an examination room. After I was asked a few questions by the nurse, she told me to remove my pants and underwear and lay faceup on the examining table, and that the doctor would be right with me. Fifteen minutes later, the doctor walked in, asked me a few more questions, and started admiring the vegetable sprouting out of my penis.

Doctor: Uh-huh.

Me: Doc, what is it?

Doctor: Hmmmm.

Me: Doc?

Doctor: Aha, hmmmm, okay, you have genital warts.

Me: *Warts?* Are you kidding me?

Doctor: No, and unfortunately it's no joke. Many kids your age are coming in with these.

Me: So how do you treat 'em?

Doctor: It's just a matter of applying a thick tarlike substance to them. I'll treat you today and then you'll need to come back every two weeks for two or three more treatments.

Me: You mean I can't get rid of these things in less than four to six weeks? That's too long!

Doctor: Well, I'm sorry, there's nothing I can do about that.

Me: Can't you give me a prescription so I can apply the medicine more often?

Doctor: No, we don't prescribe that medicine. You have to come back here for treatments. All right, I'll be back to treat you in a few moments.

Another ten minutes passed; meanwhile I was freaking out, thinking there was just no way to save the Palm Springs trip. Then the nurse walked in and placed a tray with a bunch of bottles on the table, and as she left, the doctor reentered.

> **Doctor:** Okay now, I'm going to place a drop of this [reaching for one of the bottles] on each one. It will take a few minutes to dry and then you'll be ready to go. You will need to make sure that you wash it off six to eight hours from now. Do not go to sleep tonight without washing it off! Just make sure you make an appointment for a follow-up treatment in two weeks.

So he applied the medicine to my warts, put the bottle back on the tray, and told me to wait a few minutes before getting dressed as he left the room. That's right, there I was all alone in room number 2—just me and that bottle of wart medicine. At that moment, it seemed more valuable to me than liquid gold, so I snatched it, stuck it in my sock, got dressed, and hightailed it out of there to wait for Kurt by the car. I could see the look of hopelessness on his face as he got in the car. I played along for a while before pulling the wart killer out of my sock and displaying it in front of his face. He was in shock! I told him I thought there had to be a way for us to get rid of these things quicker if we applied the medicine more often. He agreed and we called the rest of the wart squad together to give them the lowdown. We ended up divvying up the medicine among the nine of us and agreeing that we would apply it every forty-eight hours and wash it off after eight hours. As I said, nine of us divvyed it up that day, which left one of us out, Paul. Paul was a wigger before there were wiggers. He had a big nose, a big mouth, and a big cock—and an appropriately large cluster of warts on his dick, as I would find out two days later at seven thirty A.M. It was a Saturday morning, and I was in no shape to be woken up so early. That didn't matter to Paul though, as he thought nothing of squeezing his fat ass through my bedroom window that morning.

> **Paul:** Wake up, dude! I hope you saved me some of that medicine!
> **Me:** Can't we do this later?
> **Paul:** No way, bro, I gotta get to work and I don't know when I'm gonna catch you again.

Me: All right, all right—just give me a second to get my head straight.

Paul: Come on, dude, I gotta get going!

So I got up and had to find a bottle to put the shit in. I finally found one and told him to put it on every forty-eight hours. Yes, I forgot to tell him to wash it off. Of course, I didn't realize it at the time. I just went back to sleep and forgot about the whole thing. Hey, I told him I needed a second to get my head together! Now fast-forward about ten days. My warts were barely visible and most of the other guys were experiencing similar results. I was feeling confident I'd be making that trip after all and I was working out at the local gym to make sure I looked good for the Springs. Paul burst through the gym doors, ran up to me, and told me I had to follow him into the locker room. I had no idea what his problem was, but I could see he was serious, so I followed him. Once we got to the locker room, Paul walked to a secluded area and dropped his pants.

Paul: Look at my dick!

Me: What?

Paul: Dude, look at my dick! It's like it's dissolving before my eyes and it fuckin' hurts. What the fuck did you give me?

His dick really did look like it was dissolving. It was bloody and full of pus, like it was being devoured by flesh-eating bacteria.

Me: I gave you the same shit we all used! How often were you putting it on?

Paul: Every forty-eight hours, like you told me!

Me: And you washed it off after eight hours?

Paul: What are you talking about? You didn't tell me to wash it off at all, let alone after eight hours.

Me: Fuck! Sorry, dude!

I really thought that thing was going to fall off the poor guy. Thankfully, aside from a slight scar, Paul's penis was able to fully heal over time.

Unfortunately, he wasn't able to make the spring break trip, but you can bet your sweet bippy the rest of us did.

Surveys show almost every sexually active person is affected by a sexually transmitted disease at least once in their lifetime. If you read the introduction, you know that I've been personally affected, or should I say infected, three times. In all three of the cases, I will be dealing with the consequences for the rest of my life—all because I was stupid enough to have unprotected sex with women I didn't know well enough to be having unsafe sex with! Even though I will have to manage both herpes and HPV (genital warts) and have to look at my "spotted dick" every day, I still consider myself lucky considering the potential dangers of contracting and/or avoiding treatment of the variety of diseases that lurk in the genitals of people today. I'm hoping that reading this book will help you avoid many of the mistakes I've made, especially when it comes to contracting STDs. However, I am well aware that shit happens and have compiled the following information on the most common sexually transmitted diseases, including symptoms to look for and potential dangers of each:

Genital Herpes—A highly contagious virus. The symptoms of this can be so mild, many people never know they have it. Some of those infected can experience one outbreak during their lifetime, while others may suffer through regular outbreaks. In some cases, the infection can be active and contagious even when there is no visible outbreak.

> **Symptoms for Men**—Will appear irregularly and may include small red bumps, blisters, or open sores in the genital, anal, and nearby areas. Pain or itching around those same areas.
> **Symptoms for Women**—Same as men.
> **Length of time before symptoms appear**—2–14 days.
> **Danger to Men**—Aside from discomfort and inconvenience, there is no real danger, except, of course, spreading the disease to others.
> **Danger to Women**—Pregnant women risk spreading the disease to their child.
> **Treatment**—No cure. Can be suppressed with medication.

"For the first time in history, sex is more dangerous than the cigarette afterward."—Jay Leno

FACTS
- Twenty percent of the sexually active population has genital herpes.
- It is estimated that 55 million people are currently infected with genital herpes in the United States.

Gonorrhea—A bacterial infection of the genital tract.

Symptoms for Men—Yellowish discharge from penis. Burning with urination. Painful or swollen testicles.
Symptoms for Women—Yellow or bloody vaginal discharge. Burning with urination.
Length of time before symptoms appear—2–14 days.
Danger for Men—If left untreated this can lead to sterility.
Danger for Women—If left untreated this can lead to sterility.
Treatment—Antibiotics.

FACTS
- It is estimated that 650,000 Americans are infected with gonorrhea every year.
- Approximately 75 percent of all reported cases of gonorrhea are found in persons between fifteen and twenty-nine years old.

Chlamydia—A bacterial infection of the genital tract.

Symptoms for Men—Usually none. May experience burning with urination, discharge from penis, pain or swelling of testicles, or itching around the opening of the penis.
Symptoms for Women—Usually none. May experience burning

with urination, vaginal discharge, lower abdominal pain, low back pain, bleeding between menstrual periods, pain during intercourse, nausea, or fever.

Length of time before symptoms appear—5–10 days.

Danger to Men—If left untreated this can lead to urethral infection and sterility.

Danger to Women—This is the most common cause of sterility among women. Advanced stages may require the removal of the uterus, ovaries, and fallopian tubes.

Treatment—Antibiotics.

FACTS

• There are approximately three million new cases of chlamydia reported annually.

Syphilis—A bacterial infection. This disease affects your genitals, skin, and mucous membranes, but it may also affect many other areas, including the brain and heart.

Symptoms for Men—Stage 1 includes swollen, nonpainful sores called chancres. Stage 2 includes fever, rash, swollen lymph glands, sore throat, hair loss, and weight loss. Stage 3 includes paralysis, numbness, gradual blindness, dementia, and possible death.

Symptoms for Women—Same as men.

Length of time before symptoms appear—2–3 weeks.

Danger to Men—If left untreated this can cause heart disease, blindness, dementia, and death.

Danger to Women—In addition to facing the same dangers as men, pregnant women also face the added risk of exposing their unborn child to birth defects or death.

Treatment—Antibiotics.

FACTS

• Seventy-eight percent of all syphilis infections in the United States occur in African-Americans.

Crabs—Also known as pubic lice, these small parasites feed on human blood. Crabs are not the same as head and body lice. They are usually found on the pubic hair but can also be found on other parts of the body where a person has coarse hair such as armpits, eyelashes, and facial hair.

> **Symptoms for Men**—Slight to severe itching. Small red bumps in the pubic area. Pinhead-sized white eggs that stick to pubic hair and hair on the upper legs. Discolored skin patches and scratch marks in the pubic area.
> **Symptoms for Women**—Same as men.
> **Length of time before symptoms appear**—Eggs will hatch in 7–10 days
> **Danger to Men**—No severe danger unless you treasure your pubic hair more than most. They will make you itch like crazy.
> **Danger to Women**—Same as men.
> **Treatments**—Special shampoo or shaving pubic hair.

> **FACTS**
> • It is estimated that three million new cases of crabs are reported annually.

I am happy to say that I have never gotten crabs. If I was a religious man I would have to consider that a near miracle. Nevertheless, I did have an encounter with them I thought was way too close at the time. After graduating high school, my friends and I would meet for lunch at least four days per week, every week—for years. We were a tight group of eight. We were also a loose group, constantly busting chops and pulling pranks. Lunchtime seemed to be especially tempting to the jokers in our group—all of us. Whether you had to worry about the tops of the salt and pepper shakers being unscrewed or having vinegar poured in your Coke, you had to be on guard. On this particular day, it was Phil, Ron, Paul (of dissolving penis fame), and myself at Sizzler on Wilshire in Santa Monica. We had already loaded up at the all-you-can-eat salad bar and were chowing down when Paul got up to go to the bathroom. I remember immediately thinking to myself, "Dumb bastard should have finished that salad!" My mind raced through what I thought were fairly diabolical scenarios involving

Paul's neglected greens. I quickly discovered Ron and Phil were more than a few steps ahead of me. Ron reached into his backpack and pulled out what appeared to be a test tube with a capped end. They both had huge smiles on their faces as Ron moved the vial in front of my eyes for inspection. "Holy shit, what is that?" I asked. "They're crabs," he laughed. "We've been collecting them for the last six months!" I remembered hearing them bickering about passing crabs back and forth to each other (they were roommates in a small apartment) but had no idea they were keeping them as pets. There must have been close to fifty of those little critters and they were alive and kickin.' My mind hadn't fully grasped their intentions until I watched Ron remove the cap on the vial and delicately sprinkle the tiny pests over Paul's salad like Mario Batali adding a final touch of grated cheese on homemade pasta. I should have had a Guinness beer in hand because the first thought that came to mind was "Brilliant!" We needed to gather our composure quickly before Paul returned a minute or two later. Paul managed two heaping mouthfuls before Phil was squirting 7Up out his nostrils, causing both Ron and me to lose it as well. Paul knew something was up but had no idea what. He started to inspect his space. He rose up to see if he might have sat in something. He gave his salad a quick once-over with his fork and then focused on the bottom of his glass of Dr Pepper before taking a sip like the food taster for Hitler. Satisfied, he moved back to his salad. "You guys are just fucking with me," he said defiantly as he stuffed his mouth full of more "crab Louis." Then something caught his eye, causing him to move his face close to his plate—and then even closer. "What in the hell are those? They look like . . . what the fuck did you put in my salad?" Both Phil and I were cracking up, while Ron was literally rolling on the floor laughing his ass off. None of us had the ability to say a word, we were laughing so hard. Suddenly, Paul got a strange look on his face and started to rise out of his chair when he began to throw up in projectile spurts all over our table and Ron, who in turn vomited all over my feet (I was wearing flip-flops), which caused me to blow chunks all over the table. Paul was pissed, to say the least, when he found out what they put in his salad; he was still dry-heaving in the parking lot when I took off. That was the last time we would eat at Sizzler together and the closest encounter I've had with crabs to this day.

Genital Warts—Also known as human papilloma virus (HPV) and vene-real warts.

> **Symptoms for Men**—Small, flesh-colored warts that will usually appear on the penis in clusters. Itching or discomfort in the genital area. Genital warts can also develop around the scrotum, anus, mouth, or throat.
>
> **Symptoms for Women**—Same as men. However, because genital warts can grow inside the vagina or anus, these symptoms may not be visible.
>
> **Length of time before symptoms appear**—1–2 months usually, may take up to 9 months.
>
> **Danger to Men**—If left untreated, this can cause cancer of the anus and penis.
>
> **Danger to Women**—If left untreated, this can cause cervical cancer.
>
> **Treatments**—There is no cure for the virus, but the warts can be treated with injections, topical gel, or freezing. Because there is no cure for the virus, the warts can reappear over time.

FACTS

- Approximately twenty million people in the United States are currently infected with genital warts.
- Fifty to seventy-five percent of all sexually active men and women will acquire genital warts at some point in their lives.

Hepatitis B—A viral infection that affects the liver. Some people never develop signs or symptoms, while others are greatly affected by the disease.

> **Symptoms for Men**—Can include fatigue, nausea, vomiting, abdominal pain, loss of appetite, fever, dark urine, muscle or joint pain, itching, or jaundice (yellowing of skin and eyes).
>
> **Symptoms for Women**—Same as men.
>
> **Length of time before symptoms appear**—Usually 3 months, may take up to 6 months.

"If you love something, set it free. Just don't be surprised if it comes back with herpes."—Chuck Palahniuk

Danger to Men—If left untreated can cause severe liver damage, which can lead to cancer of the liver and cirrhosis.
Danger to Women—Same as men.
Treatment—No cure. Can be suppressed with medication.

FACTS
- There are approximately 100,000 new hepatitis B infections reported each year in the United States.

HIV—An infection also known as human immunodeficiency virus. HIV interferes with your body's immune system's ability to fight off the viruses, bacteria, and fungi that cause disease.

Symptoms for Men—Fever, sore throat, fatigue, or swollen lymph glands.
Symptoms for Women—Same as men.
Length of time before symptoms appear—Varies.
Danger to Men—Breakdown of the immune system and ultimately death.
Danger to Women—Same as men.
Treatment—No cure. Can be suppressed with medication.

FACTS
- It is estimated that over one million people in the United States are infected with HIV.

You want to do everything in your power to avoid catching any STDs, treatable or untreatable. Aside from always wearing condoms with new partners or abstaining from sex completely, the only other way to protect yourself is direct communication with the person you intend to have sex with. It is not considered rude or inappropriate to ask a woman about her sexual history—including STDs. Unfortunately, just because you ask doesn't mean that you're going to get honest answers, and you have to also consider the possibility that she might not even be aware that she has anything. That's why I always tell new couples that they should find a doctor or specialized testing center where both individuals can be screened for all sexually transmitted diseases together—at the same time. I say you turn it into a date by planning a meal and movie afterward. Sure, it might be an expensive day, but how much money is peace of mind worth?

Something's Fishy

Consider yourself extremely lucky if you have any level of sexual experience and haven't run into an offensively odorous vagina at least once! You know, the kind that will singe your nose hairs and make your eyes tear from a single whiff. There are many reasons why a woman can have a bad case of stank and very few things you can do about it. If I could suggest one thing, though, if you care about the woman attached to the putrid pussy, it would be to talk to her about it. The fact is, she might not have a clue that her pussy reeks in a bad way because she's had no experience with other vaginas to compare it to. You could be alerting her to a serious underlying condition. Taking it a step further, any guy can tell a woman that her coochie smells like Davey Jones' locker but it is the "dynosexual" who will have the knowledge and wherewithal to help her solve the mystery of her malodorous muff. That is why I have provided you with the following list of the nine most common causes of offensive vaginal odors.

Vaginitis—An inflammation of the vagina that results in a vaginal discharge and a foul, fishy odor. Commonly caused by thrush.

Chlamydia—Left untreated, it can result in a smelly vaginal discharge.

Poor Hygiene—Some women just don't know how to take care of their pussy! If this is the case, regular bathing, douching, and adapting to the use of baby wipes after urinating should do the trick.

Ovulation—Some women will be plagued by temporary stank when they are on the verge of their period. There's really not a lot she can do about this except for being considerate enough to provide you with a gas mask at these times.

Sperm—If you or anyone else are dumping loads of sperm into your partner and she's letting them ferment inside of her instead of rinsing herself out after each deposit, you can expect her pussy to smell like the inside of a peep show booth. Again, this is really a matter of her showering after each sex session.

Trichomoniasis—An infection caused by a microscopic parasite characterized by a smelly, heavy, yellow-green discharge.

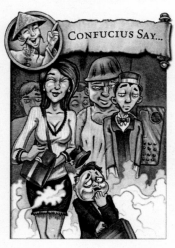

Crowded elevator smell
different to midget

Lost Tampon or Condom—Sounds funny, I know, but both actually happen to women a lot! In either case, the odor will quickly disappear once the naughty stowaway is removed.

Rectovaginal Fistula—This will make a pussy smell like ass because of an abnormal passage existing between the anal and vaginal cavities. Thankfully for both of you, this can be corrected by surgery.

Yeast Infection—Produces a cottage cheese–like discharge that will cause a starchy/old seafood type of odor.

Luckily for you, much like the clam exam mentioned in chapter 19, there is a sneaky technique you could use to try to detect an offensive vagina before it's too late. I call it the sniff test, and here's how it works.

Sniff Test—While you are making out with your prospective partner, slide your hand down to her nether region and dip your index finger into

"One of the great misconceptions is that people who have STDs know they have them . . . that is absolutely incorrect."
—Edward Nook

her pussy. Now, as you start kissing her ear, casually move that hand back up and place it near the ear you are kissing. This is the time to take a quick sniff of that finger, as she'll be so distracted by the ear play that she'll have no clue what you're up to!

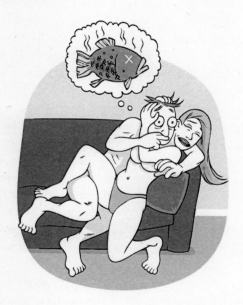

XXX Patient Beware XXX

Obviously, if you suspect you have contracted any STD, you should see a doctor immediately . . . something I have recommended a few times throughout the preceding chapters. Hence, I feel I would be doing a disservice if I did not add a caveat based on my personal experiences with doctors. First, I want to say that *most* are highly skilled, talented, intelligent, compassionate, intuitive professionals in every sense of the word. However, I need to underline the word "most" in that sentence to emphasize the fact that some are not . . . for whatever reason. Whether it's because they cheated their way through medical school, are distracted by a crumbling marriage, have a drug or alcohol problem, are too old to practice, have become fat and lazy, or really just don't give a shit—some doctors suck at being doctors! One of my personal experiences illustrates this fact best, as it left me scared, or should I say spotted, for life.

It was a gloomy morning in November of 1994. I sat in bed thinking that it must be raining STDs. After all, I had been diagnosed with herpes the previous year and there I lay in bed inspecting my penis after having been told by my girlfriend Shannon, "There's something wrong with your dick." She was right. There was something very wrong with my dick—the head of it to be exact. The skin of the head of my penis was thick, rough, and scaly. As if it were about to peel after a bad sunburn or as if my penis had actually come into contact with the sun itself. That or I was mutating into some type of mermaid. As I mumbled to myself during the inspection, Shannon added, "You should see a doctor." She was right, again. Of course, as my luck would have it I had just moved twenty-five miles away from my doctor and twenty-five miles in Los Angeles is like traveling seventy-five in most any other state. I called my dad and asked him to see if he had any friends in my area who could recommend a good doctor. He said he'd get back to me and we hung up. Having overheard the conversation, Shannon suggested her family doctor; he also happened to tend to Shannon's gynecological needs. She said he'd been taking care of her family forever—so I scheduled an appointment. When Dr. Lubit entered the examining room, I thought to myself, "I know Shannon said he'd been taking care of her family forever, but I didn't think she meant since before the Civil War." Seriously, this guy was so old he farted gold dust that could be traced back to Fort Sumter—but he was a doctor who came highly recommended by someone who I cared about. More important, by someone I knew who cared about me. This was enough for me at the time; that's why I didn't question when he diagnosed me with a yeast infection. That's why I purchased the medicine he prescribed and applied it as directed. That's why I didn't question him at my follow-up appointment when he told me, "These things take time." That's why I kept following his medical advice, with little signs of improvement in my condition, for over six months. And I can't even say it was a matter of me wising up as much as it was about breaking up . . . with Shannon that is. This meant I was single, which meant I needed to get rid of this "fish stick" and fast. So I got off my lazy ass and made the twenty-five mile trek to Dr. Rosen's. After examining me, the doc confidently told me that I did not have a yeast infection but a type of eczema. He prescribed me a cream to apply and told me to come back in two weeks. Thankfully, my condition completely cleared up within nine days . . . sort of. You see the skin on the head of my cock was back to its natural "soft as a baby's ass" smooth, but it was badly discolored. At my next appointment Dr. Rosen said he believed the discoloration was most probably a result of both the length of time it took to treat the eczema and the prolonged use of the yeast infection medicine I was originally prescribed by good old doc Lubit. Unfortunately, there was not much Dr. Rosen could do for me by then. The damage, at least aesthetically, was done.

If you have any questions now or in the future about the medical advice or treatment you or a family member is receiving, don't hesitate to seek a second opinion!

"One doctor makes work for another."—English Proverb

CHAPTER 30

The Happy Cock

Almost the entire focus of this book to this point has been on what you can do for your partner. Again, the mere fact that you're reading this book shows how important pleasuring your partner is to you. It is just as important for you to know that it is in no way selfish to expect the same consideration from your partner. A man like you deserves a reciprocal attitude and effort from your partner. Now, I'm not saying that you should expect a woman to indulge your every fantasy right off the bat. Let's face it, some of us guys have some pretty freaky fantasies. But there should be an openness, a willingness, and most importantly an eagerness to please you and explore your fantasies.

The one thing you shouldn't expect is for a woman to be able to read your mind. It is completely your responsibility to communicate your needs and desires to her. The best way to do this is obviously by initiating discussions with her. I realize that discussions about sexual matters are difficult for a lot of you. In fact, my partner Mirna and I were having some sexual communication problems at the beginning of our relationship and we decided that we would write out "What I Want in Bed" lists and exchange them. This actually worked out quite well, as it allowed us

"Having sex is like playing bridge. If you don't have a good partner, you'd better have a good hand."—Woody Allen

"Be who you are and say what you feel, because those who mind don't matter and those who matter don't mind."—Dr. Seuss

"Is life not a hundred times too short for us to stifle ourselves?"—Friedrich Nietzsche

both to be completely honest and opened up the verbal communication lines when we discussed the lists.

If you feel you are making a dynosexual-type effort and she continues to resist putting in a similar-type effort for you, well, as some of my old friends from the Bronx would say, "Time to kick the biatch to the curb!" Obviously, there are a lot of things to consider at the mention of ending a particular relationship, but ending it has to be considered, as this type of sexual neglect will fester inside you—possibly resulting in you acting out in irrational and potentially damaging ways. Remember, if you're gonna be the man who rocks her world on a regular basis, you should also expect to be treated like "the man" and have your world rocked with regularity.

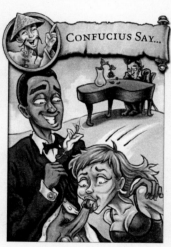

Foolish man ask for roses on piano, wise man ask for tulips on organ

THE FINAL WORD (I PROMISE!)

While this may be the end of our journey together for now, I know it is only a beginning for you. Ultimately, it is my hope this book has provided you with new perspectives, new knowledge, new techniques, new ideas, and ultimately a new level of self-confidence that gets you off to a flying start in your pursuit of sexual bliss and relationship harmony. That and knowing you enjoyed a few good laughs along the way will have made the time and effort put into this book well worth it. It's really all I need. Actually, that's not true—I would love to hear your thoughts on the book and the ways it has impacted your life, if any. Really, positive or negative . . . I'd love to hear from you! (No "poo-poo love" cracks please.)

E-mail me: seymore@earthlink.net

Twitter me: http://twitter.com/seymorebutts

A special thank-you to those who provided photos for this book:

Page 127. Picture of Ron Jeremy. Courtesy of Mike Esterman.

Page 259. Picture of We-Vibe. Courtesy of http://we-vibe.com.

Page 260. Picture of I Rub My Duckie. Courtesy of www.bigteazetoys .com.

Page 260. Picture of Liberator Wedge. Courtesy of www.liberator.com.

Page 262. Picture of Blowguard. Courtesy of www.blowguard.com.

INDEX

Note: Page numbers in *italics* refer to illustrations and page numbers followed by a *t* refer to information found in text boxes.

Also available from Vermilion

The 4-Hour Work Week

By Timothy Ferriss

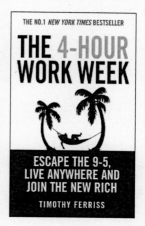

Forget the old concept of retirement and saving for the future – there is no need to wait and every reason not to. Whether your dream is escaping the rat race, experiencing first-class world travel, earning a monthly five-figure income with no management, or just living more and working less, this book is the blueprint.

In this step-by-step guide to living the life of your dreams you will learn:

- How author Timothy Ferriss went from $40,000 per year and 80 hours per week to $40,000 per month and 4 hours per week
- How to eliminate 50% of your work in 48 hours using the principles of a forgotten Italian economist
- How to exchange your career for life for short work bursts and frequent 'mini-retirements'

Discover all this and more to live the life you want – now.

£11.99   ISBN 9780091923723

Order direct from www.rbooks.co.uk

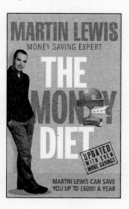